HONEY AND BEES

HONEY AND BEES

NATURE'S MAGICAL GOLDEN TREASURE

MARGARET BRIGGS

Abbeydale Press

This edition is published by Abbeydale Press, an imprint of Anness Publishing Ltd, Hermes House, 88–89 Blackfriars Road, London SE1 8HA; tel. 020 7401 2077; fax 020 7633 9499

www.annesspublishing.com

Anness Publishing has a new picture agency outlet for images for publishing, promotions or advertising. Please visit our website www.practicalpictures.com for more information.

Illustrations by Tegan Sharrard

ETHICAL TRADING POLICY

Because of our ongoing ecological investment programme, you, as our customer, can have the pleasure and reassurance of knowing that a tree is being cultivated on your behalf to naturally replace the materials used to make the book you are holding. For further information, go to www.annesspublishing.com/trees

A CIP catalogue record for this book is available from the British Library.

Previously published as *Honey and its Many Health Benefits*

THE AUTHOR

Margaret Briggs was a teacher for 30 years, working in Kent, North Yorkshire and Sussex, UK. Since leaving teaching she has had more time for gardening and cooking, and has embarked on a second career as a freelance writer, researcher and editor, alongside her writer husband, Lol. The couple now live in south-west France where they renovated a dilapidated house. The house is now restored and Margaret and Lol divide their time between Sussex and the Gironde, with two contrasting gardens to develop.

PUBLISHER'S NOTE

CONTENTS

Introduction

HONEY: A MODERN HEALER

Honey bees have been around longer than humans.
We know that thanks to fossil evidence from 150 million
years ago. But from the earliest times man has used this
natural product to nourish, heal, purify and protect. It is
well known that prehistoric man worshipped the sun as
the supreme giver and sustainer of life. How many of us
are aware, however, that honey figured in the rituals of
the Babylonians and Assyrians? They used to pour honey
on the foundations and walls of their temples. Similar
customs existed among the ancient Egyptians and, across
the other side of the world, the Incas. Hindus and
Persians used honey in religious services, considering it a
sacred, divine food and cleanser.

Some of these ancient rituals still exist today in parts of
Africa and honey collection still has certain time
constraints relating to ancient beliefs.

Although early man didn't know about the antibacterial
qualities of honey and the benefits of eating honey for
health and energy, he knew that he liked the sweet taste
and that it was produced by some alchemy involving
bees. It was the only sweetener readily available until
fairly recent times. Victorian cooks like Mrs Beeton
discovered that loaf sugar was much more convenient for
a number of recipes. Apart from honey as a sweetener,
there are innumerable other benefits to be obtained from
bees, including the production of wax for candles and
fermented honey to produce an alcoholic drink. The word
'mead' and its derivations in several languages mean
various things connected with honey. Poets waxing lyrical
through the ages have come to use the taste of honey as
a metaphor for love, and generations of children have
learned to love 'silly old bears' that get stuck in sticky
situations because of it.

Cleopatra knew a thing or two about beauty and used to
bathe in honey and milk to keep her skin smooth. Modern

beauty treatments still use honey to enhance the appearance of the skin.

This book sets out to entertain the interested armchair enthusiast, rather than to inform on the finer points of beekeeping, honey types and therapies. Having said that, I hope you will be as fascinated as I am by the sheer versatility of this natural product.

Know Your Bees

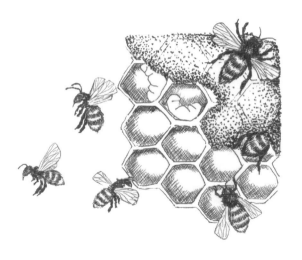

APOIDEA: A SUPERFAMILY

Bees belong to the insect family Hymenoptera, which also includes ants, wasps and sawflies. Hymenoptera are important to man as pollinators of wild and cultivated plants. These insects have always had a bad time with many humans, who only see in them the potential for nasty stings and ant invasions, but they can also be parasites of destructive insects and makers of honey.

The 20,000 or so species of bees so far identified are found virtually worldwide. The only places you won't find them are at very high altitudes, in Polar regions and on some oceanic islands. The greatest number of species is found in warm, subtropical and tropical areas. Bees range in size from 2 mm (0.08 in) in length to a rather scary 4 cm (1.6 in) long. Many bees are black or brown, but others incorporate bright yellow, red and metallic green or blue.

Like other hymenoptera, bees have four wings and a narrow waist that separates the abdomen from the thorax. The mouth is modified to make it a sucking type. The egg-laying organ, or ovipositor, is often very long and is modified for piercing, sawing or stinging. The sex of the insect is dependent upon whether the egg was fertilised: if fertilised, they become female and if unfertilised they remain male. Most bees have specialised, feathery body hairs to help with the collection of pollen.

There are 11 families of bees, distinguished by subtle differences in wing veins and by the structure of the mouth and other minor characteristics. The bees in each family have other distinguishing features, including body hair, the length of the tongue, and the form of pollen-carrying equipment.

CELLOPHANE BEES are fairly hairless bees with short, forked tongues. They look more like wasps than bees and are considered the most primitive bees. They line their nest tunnels and chambers for the young with a secretion that hardens into a cellophane-like skin. They carry pollen on leg hairs or internally in a stomach-like crop.

MINING BEES make soil nests of many branching chambers, each ending in one or more cells. They can be solitary or communal, living in separate nests but close to each other. They carry pollen on body and leg hairs.

LEAFCUTTER BEES and *MASONRY BEES* belong to a family of long-tongued bees that have pollen-carrying hairs on the underside of the abdomen. Some are used in agriculture to pollinate crops.

SWEAT BEES are generally small, dark-coloured bees with little hair. They usually nest in the ground but may live in societies in which related bees help each other. Pollen is carried on brushy areas near the base of the legs and on body hairs.

DIGGER and *CARPENTER BEES* are fast-flying and may nest in the ground on their own or in dense clusters. They are excellent pollinators of many plants. Carpenter bees nest in plant stems. Some can excavate burrows in solid wood. They range in size from 0.6 cm (0.2 in) to 2.5 cm (1 in) in length and are darkish green and blue in colour.

HONEY BEES and their close relatives are the most familiar bees. These bees make intricate nests and live in complex societies. The pollen-carrying structure is a smooth, bristle-surrounded area on the middle of the hind leg, known as a pollen basket or corbicula. Close relatives are the orchid bee, bumble bee and stingless bee. Honey bees and stingless bees commonly hoard large quantities of honey which has, for centuries, been a characteristic exploited by man.

POLLINATION

Bees, along with other hymenoptera, are the most important pollinating insects. Their mutual dependency with flowering plants makes for a symbiotic relationship, where each is benefiting the other. Many plants cannot reproduce without the help of a specific species of insect. Bees are dependent on pollen as a protein source and harvest nectar as an energy source.

Social adult females collect pollen mainly to feed their larvae. The pollen lost in going from flower to flower is important to plants because some pollen lands on the pistils or reproductive organs of other flowers of the same species, resulting in cross-pollination.

BEE SOCIETIES

SOLITARY BEES

Most species of bees are solitary, which means that each female makes her own nest. They are short-lived as adults, having grown through the stages of egg, lava and pupa before attaining adulthood.

ANTHOPHORINAE

This group includes bees that nest in the ground, often in large colonies, such as miner bees, digger bees and cuckoo bees. These are primitive bees and like their relatives, the wasps, they are solitary. Each female makes a burrow, in which she constructs earthen chambers for her young. Pollen moistened with nectar or oil is deposited into individual cells until enough food has accumulated to provide for the larva until it reaches full size. The female then lays an egg on the pollen mass and seals the cell before constructing another one.

CLEPTOPARASITIC BEES

This subgroup of parasitic or cuckoo bees do not forage or make their own nests but use the nests of other bee species to provide for their young. They invade the nests of solitary bees and hide their eggs in the chambers prepared by the host before the host can lay her own eggs. The chambers are then sealed. The young parasitic bees then prosper on the prepared food that had been so carefully left by the host. The other eggs or larvae of the host are then killed by the parasitic bees or the larvae. Female parasitic bees don't have pollen baskets or pollen brushes, as they don't need to forage for food for their young.

SOCIAL BEES or APINAE

This is the group that includes the social bees, including honey bees and bumble bees. There are also communal bees, where several females of the same generation use the same nest, each making cells to house their own eggs, larvae and pupae. Some are semi-social, living in colonies of two to seven worker bees with a queen. About 1,000 such species form colonies that die out in the autumn, with only the queens surviving the winter.

Bumble bees come into this category. The best-known groups of social bees live in large colonies of two generations of mothers and daughters, with males playing no part in the organisation of the colony. They only mate with the queens. Since this book is about honey, the societies described from now on relate to honey bees.

HONEY BEE COLONIES

A colony of honey bees functions more or less as a single organism. This is no mean feat, given the knowledge that a colony can be made up of a queen bee, up to 60,000 undeveloped females and up to 1,000 drone or male bees. Only the females have a sting. Of course if you are worried about being stung, or have an allergic reaction to bee stings, this is not good news, given the ratio of male to female bees.

Honey bee colonies collect a variety of matter to enable life in the colony to run smoothly. This includes:

NECTAR, which is converted into honey. When collected from blossoms, stems and leaves, the nectar contains 50 to 80% water, but by the time it is converted into honey it will be only 16 to 18% water.
HONEYDEW, stored as honey. This is a sweet liquid collected from other insects such as aphids and caterpillars.
POLLEN, a dust-like male element from the anthers of flowers. Pollen provides the protein for rearing young bees.
PROPOLIS, a resinous material collected from the buds of trees, which is used for sealing cracks in the hive, in addition to covering unwanted objects which the bees can't remove from the hive. As well as defensive and protective properties, it is also known to have many beneficial medical uses. See the section on benefits to health for more details.
WATER, for air-conditioning the hive and to dilute the honey the bees consume.

HIVES

Since the seventeenth century man has been aware of the
basic life cycle of bees, their production of honey and
how to control them with smoke. Given this knowledge
it became easier for people to farm the bees to produce
honey by assisting the formation of the hive through a
wax comb foundation.

Bees produce tiny flakes of wax which is secreted from
the underside of the abdomen. They use these flakes to
mould beeswax into honeycomb. This is made up of thin-
walled, back-to-back hexagons to form cells. The cells in
the hive are used for a variety of purposes, depending on
the need of the colony. They can be used for storing
honey or pollen or for the queen to lay eggs in, one per
cell. Generally the honey is stored towards the top of the
comb and pollen in cells closer to the area where bees
develop from eggs, called the brood nest. The
temperature here must remain at about 34°C (93°F),
whatever the weather conditions may be like outside the
nest. A colony can survive in temperatures of 49°C
(120°F) as long as there is water for the air-conditioning.
If the temperature falls below 14°C (57°F) the bees stop
flying and form a tight cluster to insulate the brood and
conserve energy. Bees can survive for weeks on end in
temperatures of −46°C (−51°F), which must make them
Olympian survivors.

SWARMING

The cycle of renewal starts with swarming, when the
colony is becoming overcrowded. When there are
plentiful supplies of flowers and pollen in summer the
queen lays more eggs and honey is built up in the combs.
With the emergence of a large number of young bees the
hive rapidly becomes overcrowded and there is no room
for the queen to lay more eggs. Worker bees then choose
about a dozen larvae that would become worker bees
without further intervention, but instead they feed them
with a white food called royal jelly. This is produced by
the workers from a gland in their heads. Having been fed
copious amounts of royal jelly the larvae develop instead
into virgin queens, but just before these queens emerge

the mother queen will leave the hive with the swarm. All of the departing bees are provided with supplies of honey.

Swarming usually takes place on a hot day. Between 5,000 and 25,000 worker bees (about half the colony) will swirl out into the air. If you haven't ever experienced a swarm of bees it's difficult to describe the dense, noisy cloud that accompanies this flight. It can be quite alarming and became an almost annual occurrence at the rural primary school where I used to teach. They usually made for the Victorian roof of the school hall. Bees have been known to alight on trees, fire hydrants and cars as well as rooftops. The bees form a tight, protective cluster around the queen while a few scouts go out looking for a new home. When this has been found the swarm takes to the air again and swirls along in a mass. See below to find out how they all know where to go.

WHO'S QUEEN?
Meanwhile, back at the original colony, the first queen to emerge after the departure of the mother queen with the swarm gets to work on destroying the other young queens. If two emerge together they will fight to the death. After about a week the new queen will take her nuptial flight, frequently mating with more than one drone while in the air. After perhaps another couple of flights she will start egg laying and will rarely leave the colony again, except with a swarm. There will be enough sperm stored in her sperm pouch to fertilise all the eggs she will lay for the rest of her life, which may be up to

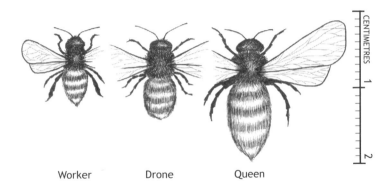

Worker   Drone   Queen

CENTIMETRES 1 2

five years. As for the drones she mated with, they die in the act of mating. It is the queen who decides whether or not she needs drones or workers, and when she lays eggs she controls the sperm duct by contracting or relaxing a muscular ring.

THE EGG STAGE

A bee egg is about half the size of a grain of rice and only takes the queen a few seconds to lay. She can lay up to 1,900 eggs a day. Each egg is attached to the wall of the cell by a strand of mucus. During the next three days the nervous system, digestive organs and outer covering of the bee will form. The egg remains in an upright position for the first three days, then leans over on to its side, when it hatches as a larval bee, without legs, wings, antennae or eyes.

THE LIFE CYCLE OF THE HONEY BEE

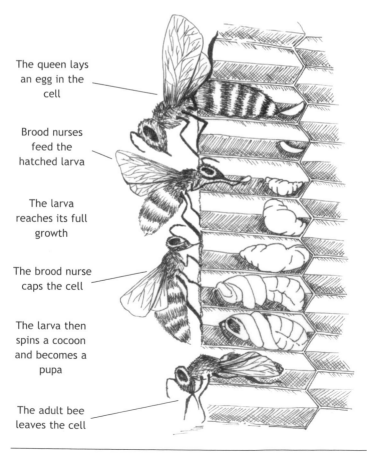

The queen lays an egg in the cell

Brood nurses feed the hatched larva

The larva reaches its full growth

The brood nurse caps the cell

The larva then spins a cocoon and becomes a pupa

The adult bee leaves the cell

LARVAL STAGE

The larva now looks like a rice grain with a mouth and that's all it needs for the moment, as its function is to do nothing but eat and grow. At this stage the larva will be visited up to 1,300 times a day by the brood nurses who feed it 'bee bread', made from honey, pollen and secretions from the brood nurses (see below). Richer food, royal jelly, is only given to potential queen larvae. As the larva grows it passes through five stages, shedding a skin after each of the first four stages. It has 13 sections to its body and a small head. The stomach is well developed, as is the honey stomach or crop, and there are depressions where the antennae will grow. The mandibles, maxillae and duct of the silk gland are developed. After six days the larva reaches the final stage, where the cell is capped by a worker bee and the larva spins a cocoon.

PUPA STAGE

Queens hatch from pupae after eight days, whereas worker bees and drones take longer to pupate. A worker emerges after 12 days and a drone, 14 days. A queen or a drone will weigh 200 mg and a worker about half that amount.

DRONES

The sex of the offspring is determined by the queen. If she does not fertilise the eggs she lays they become males or drones. Drones are only reared when there is plenty of nectar and pollen. They live for a few weeks, but are the first to get the elbow when conditions deteriorate, for example in the autumn. They are virtual parasites: the only duty of the drone is to mate with the queen, so if she's not in the mood for mating, there's no need to give the drones houseroom and feed them. Simple economics really!

WORKER BEES

Tasks in the beehive are allocated by age. Worker bees do all of the work except egg laying. Larvae are completely dependent on the continuous care of adults. On the day a bee emerges as an adult this female worker starts to carry out waste, clean the cells and line them with a new disinfectant material ready for new eggs. After about three days the young bee becomes a brood nurse. She provides the larvae with pollen and honey. On the sixth day she also starts to feed the larvae with special food which she produces from a pharyngeal gland. On Day 16 the bee becomes active in secreting wax to build the honeycomb. Soon after this she makes her first flight outside to find her way around. On Day 20 she starts guard duty, serving on the entrance to the hive. Finally she becomes a collector bee and remains in this job until her death. Worker bees live for about six weeks normally, but may live for several months if they emerge in the autumn and spend the winter in the hive.

ANATOMY OF THE HONEY BEE

Insects have three body regions:
the head, thorax and abdomen.

THE STRUCTURE OF THE HONEY BEE

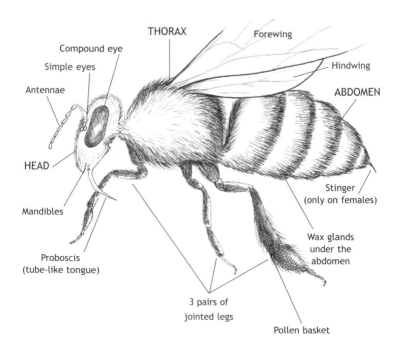

HEAD

Two *antennae* rise from the centre of the head. These are important sensory organs and are set in small sockets so that they can move freely. The tiny hairs on each antenna are responsive to touch and smell.

A bee has five eyes, consisting of a pair of *compound eyes*, made up of numerous hexagonal facets, and three simple eyes on top of its head which are sensitive to light. Bees don't have particularly sharp vision, however, and it seems that the patterns of the flowers attract the bees rather than their geometric shapes. The bee is capable of sensing ultraviolet radiation but is blind to red light. This means that white flowers appear to be coloured to a bee and certain colour combinations invisible to humans are of particular interest to bees. Some flowers that appear entirely yellow to humans appear to bees as only yellow around the nectar source, thereby directing the bees more efficiently. Bees use their eyes for orientation from the hive to food sources very effectively. A keen sense of smell ensures that all members of the colony have the same odour. Guards at the entrance smell each bee that seeks to enter. The queen bee also secretes her own smell, so that as long as she produces her scent no other queen can be produced.

The *proboscis* is simply a long, thin, hairy tongue that acts like a straw to get liquid to the mouth. The flexible tip makes a lapping motion and when feeding has finished the proboscis is drawn up behind the head.

The *mandibles* are pincer-like jaws with a chewing mouthpart. These are used to fight, to mould wax and to cut through flower tissue to get to the nectar. The *maxillae* are a second pair of feelers used for food handling and sensing.

THORAX

The thorax is the anchor for three pairs of legs as well as two pairs of wings. *Pollen baskets* are located on the hind legs. The forelegs are antennae cleaners.

ABDOMEN

The digestive tracts of honey bees are similar to most other *hymenoptera*. The oesophagus enlarges near the stomach to form a crop or honey *stomach*, where an adult honey bee can carry up to 75 mg of nectar — about a third of the entire body weight of the bee. The *sting* is the same structure as the egg-laying organ in other insects but has been modified in honey bees to eject venom. Only females have a sting. When not in use it is pulled back into the abdomen. There will be more about bee stings later.

DANCING BEES

Highly integrated communities like bee colonies need a sophisticated method of passing information from one to another. Bees have their own unique system of letting each other know about food supplies, possible new homes, etc. After a bee has found food she returns to the hive, fully laden with nectar and pollen. She then proceeds to tell the rest of the workers where to find the source of the new food. The information she relates includes the location, quantity and quality of the nectar. Information on the species of plant is conveyed by means of the smell of the flower which is stuck to the bee's body. Other bees sense this information through their antennae.

The bee tells her sisters about the quality and quantity of food through a series of lively dance movements. The rhythm of the dance explains where the source can be found and the closer the food, the greater the number of cycles performed. If the food is near the hive she performs a round dance. If the source is to be found further away, i.e. more than 80 m (260 ft), she will perform a tail-waggling dance. Ten cycles performed in 15 seconds means that the food is 100 m (330 ft) away, whereas if the source is 10,000 m away (33,000 ft) she will perform only one cycle of movements in the same time. The bee measures the distance in terms of how much energy is used in travelling.

The dance transmits information on direction as well as distance by using the sun and gravity. During flight the bee works out the angle between the sun and the line of flight. By dancing on the honeycomb she describes the angle needed to locate the food. Upward tail wagging means 'go towards the sun', whereas a downward run means 'fly away from the sun'. A run 45 degrees left shows the source to be on that plane. Of course, since the position of the sun changes throughout the day the bees must change the angle of the dance as well. If the sun is covered by cloud or a tall building, mountain or trees, the bee will use knowledge of polarisation by analysing the intensity of light.

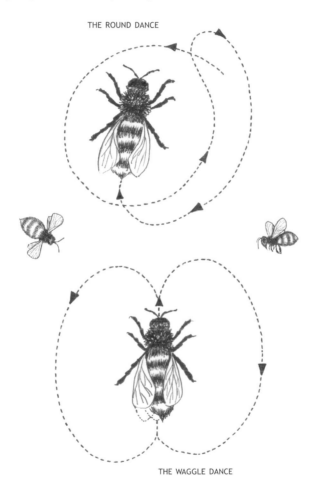

THE ROUND DANCE

THE WAGGLE DANCE

Tail waggling is also performed when the swarm is looking for a new home. When the scouts return to the queen they describe the possible new home in the same way.

The History behind Honey

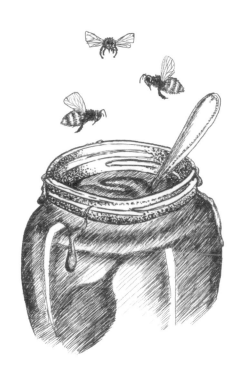

CHINESE PUZZLE

There are fossilised remains of honey bees dating back 150 million years, and the earliest records of bee-keeping date back to 7000 BC. Chemical analysis of the evidence of pottery fragments from jars unearthed in the Neolithic village of Jiahu in the Henan province in Northern China have revealed that a fermented drink made from rice, honey and fruit was being produced as early as 9,000 years ago. Jiahu must have been quite a trendsetting place in its time, as early examples of musical instruments and farmed rice were also discovered there.

Archaeologists have discovered pottery vessels from Neolithic times which are very similar to those found from much later, suggesting that there was a need for storage of beverages much earlier than previously thought. Given also the knowledge that honey bees are one of the oldest forms of animal life known to exist in that period and that Neolithic man gathered and ate honey and honeycombs, it's not surprising that the only available sweetener was used in drinks. This was about the same time as barley beer and wine from grapes were being made in the Middle East.

In Spain discoveries have been made of paintings, said to be around 7,000 years old, showing the process of bee-keeping.

THE ANCIENT EGYPTIAN BEE-KEEPERS

The Ancient Egyptians used honey nearly 4,000 years ago to sweeten their food. It was highly valued because of its therapeutic qualities, and honey played an important role in the cultural life of the people as it was associated with both birth and death. The consumption of high energy honey, both before conception and to promote fertility, was as important as the inclusion of honey as an ingredient in embalming fluid.

CRY ME A HIVER

The earliest records of bee-keeping in hives for honey production are attributed to the Egyptians and date back to 2400 BC. The hives shown in pictures in tombs consisted of woven baskets covered with clay, similar to those still in use today in the Sudan. Cylindrical hives made of clay were also used. The centre of bee-keeping seems to have been the cultivated lands of Lower Egypt, where the bee was chosen as a symbol for the country and one of the pharaoh's titles was 'Bee King'. This relates to the myth of the god Re, whose tears, as he wept, fell to the ground and became bees. The bees began to be active on all the flowers belonging to the earth. So honey was created from the tears of the god.

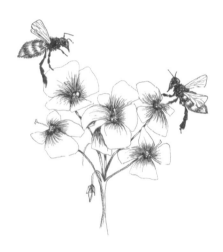

FREE-RANGE HONEY

Apparently nomadic Egyptians kept bees as well, using the honey as part of green eye paint. Itinerant bee-keepers living by the Nile loaded their hives onto boats to carry upriver in the spring and then followed the flowering of plants gradually northwards. Wild honey seems to have been in even greater demand. Honey hunters were protected by royal archers while searching the wadis for colonies of bees. Temples kept bees for offerings to the gods as well as for producing medicines and ointments. The Egyptians knew about applying honey to wounds to aid healing, even if they didn't understand the antibacterial and fungicidal qualities of the product. The demand for honey was greater than the production, so along with other luxury goods, it was imported from elsewhere, including Canaan, the area today encompassing Israel and Palestine and referred to in the Old Testament as the land of milk and honey.

MONEY HONEY

The Egyptians valued honey so highly that they frequently offered it to their gods and high-born members of society. Honey was only available to rich people, the poorer members of society having to make do with dates and fruit juice to sweeten their food. It was also used as a type of currency and was fed to animals considered sacred in Egyptian culture. During later times around the birth of Jesus, there are reports of sacred animals receiving meals of a mash of wheat flour prepared with honey pastries, honey mead, goose meat and other birds. These sacred animals included the ram in Mendes, a lion in Leontopolis and a crocodile in the Lake of Moeris. Herodotus, the 5th century BC Greek historian, known as the Father of History, tells of sacrificial animals also being prepared with honey. A bullock would have the entrails removed as well as the legs, shoulders and neck. The body cavity was then filled with consecrated loaves of bread and honey, along with figs, raisins and spices which included frankincense and myrrh. The whole sacrifice was then covered with oil to preserve it.

Remnants of papyrus have been found with lists of food including wine, bread, pickled fish, honey and vinegar for trade, showing what a healthy diet the Ancient Egyptians enjoyed. Evidence from tombs shows that they had over 30 different types of bread, including the round, flat loaf now called pita bread. Sweetened doughs were made by combining honey with dates and other fruit, nuts and spices.

EGYPTIAN WAX

As well as making wide use of honey for culinary and medicinal purposes the Egyptians also used wax extensively. Beeswax has been found in association with boat building, mummification, paints and metal casting. It served as a medicine and, when mixed with pulverised stone, it provided a means of sticking razors to handles.

Wax was also used to keep wigs in good condition and plaits in place, and for making writing tablets during the reign of Ptolemy.

WHICH DOCTOR?

Don't imagine that sticking pins into wax models was a more modern invention; ritual figurines were made from wax which could then be destroyed by fire or force. Spells and incantations were written or drawn on papyrus with green ink and performed over the figures to enfeeble the limbs of enemies or to bewitch them so that they could easily be caught and killed. Wax also appears on lists of offerings for festivals, along with bread, beer and wine, showing the importance of this commodity.

THE ANCIENT GREEKS

Ancient Greek civilisation offered honey to the spirits of the dead and, like the Egyptians, believed that it was part of the staple diet of their gods. Zeus, the king of the Greek gods, was fed nectar from queen bees during his childhood and honey became known as ambrosia, the food of the gods. Honey was thought to prolong life and give strength. As a child Jupiter was hidden on Crete from his father, who was full of envy and out to get him. While in hiding, Jupiter was fed honey and milk, which made him strong enough to seize the throne from his father when he grew up.

NECK SOME NECTAR AND STOP THE COFFIN

The Ancient Greeks also realised that honey had pharmaceutical values and medicinal qualities, and was therefore also an important, nutritious food for humans. Mead was first made by the Greeks as an alcoholic beverage and called the nectar of the gods. Honey was a symbol of blessedness and happiness to the Greeks and honey mixed with blood became the highest form of offering to the gods. It played an important part in festivals, especially funeral ceremonies. Later, pagans also used honey, placing it inside coffins and on graves.

Hippocrates, the father of modern medicine, promoted the usefulness of honey in relieving a number of ailments, and Aristotle, both a philosopher and scientist, thought that honey was good for the digestion, leading to a longer, healthier life. Pythagoras also affirmed, when he reached 90, that he owed his great age to honey; he thought he would otherwise have died when ill at the age of 50. Democritus is also said to have prolonged his life by eating honey, so that his daughters could enjoy the festival associated with the goddess Ceres. Greek mythology tells that Eros, the god of love, dipped his arrows in honey before wreaking havoc with humans' love lives. The Roman version, Cupid, repeated this practice.

HONEY ROMAN EMPIRE
During Roman times the spread of apiculture, or bee-keeping, became a feature of life throughout the Roman Empire. Apiaries became widespread and guaranteed that honey harvesting flourished across the Roman world.

LET IT BEE
With the establishment of Christianity came a greater demand for honey and also for beeswax. The early Christians had special regard for honey which had a deeply spiritual association. It was given to newly christened converts as a symbol of renovation. In later times monks and clergy kept bees to ensure that there was a regular supply of beeswax for candles as well as for writing, sealing and protecting art works. Honey was also used in some recipes for ink. This involved mixing albumen, or egg white, with soot and blending it with honey to form a smooth paste.

In feudal Russia people who were bee-keepers were called bortniks. From the 13th to the 15th centuries these bortniks enjoyed higher status than other peasants. Bortniks, who gradually became free people, lived on the forest edges where the bees belonging to noblemen were kept, enjoying some privilege by working for themselves and living on the products produced.

AMBROSIA OR ANGELS' DELIGHT?

The first recorded introduction of honey bees from Europe to South America was in 1530. The Spanish invaders of Mexico and Central America, however, were surprised to see that the production of honey and bee-keeping were already long established. The bees were stingless and about the same size as domestic flies. Honey was discovered in the hollows of dead trees, in the ground or attached to branches of trees. Native Indians also supplied them with earthenware jars and logs in which to nest. The honey produced by these 'Angelitos' or little angels was thin but much preferred by the Indians, after the white man's bees were introduced, for its beneficial qualities.

Honey played an important part in the lives of the ancient Mayan and Aztec civilisations. Conquered tribes had to pay tributes of honey, as recorded in one instance when 700 pottery jars of honey were paid to Montezuma, the Aztec emperor of Mexico. These tribes were then allowed to keep producing honey and pottery as two main occupations and sources of future revenue. Mexican Indians prayed to their bee god for plenty of honey. A number of folk stories connected with the search for honey are very similar to those told by Russian, Hindu, African and East Indian people.

When European settlers from Britain, Spain and Holland reached North America in 1638, the new colonists brought European honey bees with them. Native people called the new species of bee 'white man's fly'. The settlers developed a wide range of applications, including use of honey in cement, preserving fruit and in making furniture polish and varnish.

NO TASTE OF HONEY . . .

The introduction of bees from Florida to Cuba didn't go too smoothly in 1764, when the planters of sugar cane annihilated the bees because they were 'stealing' the sugar cane. Bees were first introduced to Argentina around 1840, to Brazil in 1848 and to Chile and Peru in 1857. Once sugar cane became available, honey became less popular for sweetening food, but that doesn't mean that honey was less important.

. . . BUT A MOVABLE FEAST

If the experiences of the people of Hawaii are anything to go by, the introduction of bees was not always simply a matter of ordering a hive. In their case it took some years and several failed attempts. In August 1851 on the island of Oahu, a committee was appointed to bring the first honey bees into Hawaii. A hive was shipped from Boston to Honolulu in 1852 but unfortunately, as the ship passed through the tropics, the increase in temperature melted the honeycomb and killed the honey bees. Another colony ordered from New Zealand was never shipped, due to an apparent misunderstanding. A second attempt to ship bees from the US mainland was made in 1853, with two hives, one of which was packed in ice. These hives arrived in poor condition; the bees survived for a short time, then died out. The committee then made the generous public offer of ten dollars reward to the person who could bring honey bees to the island. It was not until October 1857 that three hives of German dark bees were shipped to Honolulu. The trip took 18 days and this time the colonies survived the journey in good condition, to be purchased for the princely sum of 100 dollars each. The hives thrived and by the following year the original hives had increased to nine colonies. Such was the importance of bees to the island, not only for honey production but also to stimulate the sugar cane industry.

WAX AND TAX

It wasn't just the Ancients who used honey for trade and payment of dues. The *Domesday Book* contains a number of references to hives and honey being used in payment by towns throughout the kingdom. In the 11th century German beer was sweetened with honey, and lords' feudal dues were paid in honey and wax.

People knew long ago that bees produce honey, that they sting and that they increase their numbers by swarming. By the 17th century man had learned the value of smoke to control bees and had developed the screen veil to protect against stings. The following two centuries yielded some major discoveries on which modern bee-keeping is based. These included the following:

- The mystery of the queen bee as the mother of nearly all the other occupants of the hive.
- The development of unfertilised eggs into adult drones.
- Mating techniques of the queen.
- The rearing of a new queen by the other bees if the old queen disappeared.
- The invention of movable frame hives.
- Understanding how to divide a colony instead of waiting for swarming.
- The development of a wax comb foundation as a starter comb, so that bees could build straight combs which are easier to handle.
- The discovery that honey can be centrifuged from combs, which can then be reused.

Work on bee diseases and their control and an understanding of pollen in producing the strongest colonies have also increased production and led to modern, commercial organisation of the honey industry.

ANTIPODES HAD NO BEES!
Bees were introduced to Australia in 1822 and New Zealand in 1839. It seems surprising, given that some of the most famous honeys in the world come from these countries, that there were no indigenous species of bee before these dates.

HONEY TRAP — MONEY TRAP
Few countries held honey in higher esteem than France. As in other countries in Europe in feudal times, honey was used in France as a source of tax revenue, with lords able to collect from honey hunters and keepers of beehives. A proportion of honey and wax had to be given up. In 1791, during the French Revolution, the government of the day demanded a record of all hives, resulting in many being destroyed rather than the owners paying more tax. For a long time after, apiculture was sadly neglected.

A bizarre law was passed in 1934 whereby a bee-keeper was assessed for tax on agricultural rates if the bees were fed on his own property, but on a higher rate if the bees buzzed off to a neighbour's property, when the honey could be taxed as a non-commercial business. Imagine being a tax inspector! This law is obviously obsolete now:

'last year I visited a local producer of acacia honey in South West France, near where I live. The bees had been sent out to forage on the numerous acacia trees in the local area and I don't think they had the owner's permission somehow.'

The island of Corsica is still renowned for its honey, but back in the times of Roman occupation its people had to contribute 200,000 lb of wax in yearly tribute. This means that the bees must have produced over a million lb of honey a year.

MEAD
Any history of honey would be incomplete without consideration of mead, probably the oldest known fermented drink. The very word mead is possibly related to the various words for honey found in different languages. We don't know who first brewed mead, but it has been around for several thousand years. There are reports of King Solomon and the Queen of Sheba being toasted with mead at their wedding, and mead is the national drink of Ethiopia, where it is known as T'ej and has been produced for 5,000 years.

Perhaps the discovery was made after someone found some honey in an old bee-hive or tree trunk that had been diluted with rainwater and fermented by wild yeasts which exist all around. Whatever the origin, fermentation served as purification for unsafe water supplies.

DROP OF MEAD, HENRY HONEY?
Mead brewing became a tradition in northern Europe, in the areas that did not support vines for wine growing. Hence the Vikings, Saxons and Celts were all notable imbibers of mead. England's history of mead making is long but not well recorded. After the dissolution of the

monasteries by Henry VIII, the monks who had been skilled in bee-keeping, honey and mead production became scattered so that brewing only survived as a small-scale cottage industry, then beer took over.

Early meads were heavily spiced, to cover up unpleasant flavours caused by the fermentation by wild yeasts. This meant that fermentation was rather hit and miss before Pasteur's work in 1857, when he discovered that the process was caused by a living micro-organism.

LOVING CUP – KEEP IT UP!

Many traditions associated with honey and mead originate from Scandinavia, where mead is the beverage of love. The word honeymoon relates to the revelry attached to wedding celebrations by the Vikings. If you think modern wedding celebrations are long and costly, spare a thought for the poor hosts in days gone by. The guests danced and drank until the mead and ale ran out, which was traditionally a lunar month after the nuptials. If the drinks ran out early there may have been ugly scenes! Drinking mead was also important for fertility and the birth of sons. This was very important when male offspring accounted for great status in warring clans and factions. The Vikings also thought that drinking mead for a month after the wedding would result in the first born child being male. Special cups were used which were handed down through the generations, suggesting some magical powers for producing male babies. Successful male births were a further excuse for a great knees-up, and, with the alcoholic content of mead being around 12%, there would have been quite a party. The maker of the mead also had his reputation to maintain and was congratulated on the couple's success along with the groom, who could then boast of his virility and power.

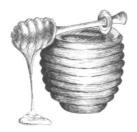

Bee-keeping
for
'Beeginners'

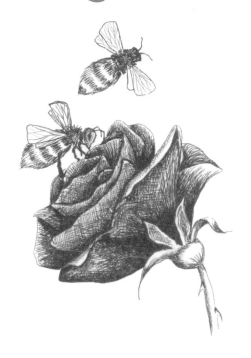

For much of this section I am indebted to Graham Law, a bee-keeper and mine of information. I've found his excellent website (*www.beeginners.info*) both informative and entertaining and, with his permission, have drawn extensively on his knowledge. This book doesn't attempt to go into great detail on bee-keeping, but the process is a fascinating one which is worthwhile exploring. Graham can tell you everything you want to know!

HIVES
The 'classic' picturesque terraced beehive frequently seen in the UK is usually the WBC (William Broughton Carr 1890) hive. This is a double-walled hive, utilising inner boxes and outer covers, called 'lifts'. Most hobbyists in the UK use the single-walled British National Hive, which uses the same internal frames as the WBC but has fewer components to move during routine inspections.

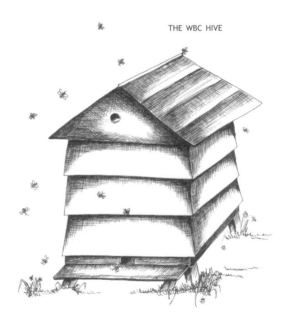

THE WBC HIVE

The other styles that are used in the UK and are common elsewhere are the Langstroth and the Commercial. Both are single-walled and larger than the British National. In the north of the UK, especially Scotland, the Smith hive is popular. This is a nice compromise and uses the same frames as the National except that the frame lugs, the bits that stick out at the top of the frame, are shorter. Professionally made equipment, especially if made from cedar wood, will last a lifetime and the manufacturers are well geared up for mass production.

LOCATION, LOCATION

The 'ideal' location for a beehive is on the edge of trees on a south-facing slope with no public access or nearby paths, out of reach of cattle or horses. It should also have easy access by vehicle. Bees don't like being sited in an area that is damp, such as in the middle of a wood or in a hollow. They like somewhere that is well ventilated but not in a wind tunnel. On the edge of a coppice is ideal. The hives should be on stands about 300—400 mm (12—15 in) high and allow air movement beneath them. Hives are set no closer than 1 m (3 ft) apart and the entrances must not be in a straight line, as this will just encourage bees to drift into other hives, a trait that will cause disease to spread easily and tend to weaken some colonies in favour of others.

HOW HONEY IS MADE

Bees take nectar, the sweet sticky substance exuded by most flowers and some insects, and mix it with enzymes from glands in their mouths. This nectar and enzyme mix is stored in hexagonal wax honeycomb until the water content has been reduced to about 17%. When this level is reached the cell is capped over with a thin layer of wax to seal it until the bees need it to feed on. This capping indicates to the bee-keeper that the honey is ready for harvesting. Capped honey will keep almost indefinitely.

Here's the science:

SUCROSE (NECTAR) + INVERTASE (BEE ENZYME) = FRUCTOSE + GLUCOSE (HONEY)

The queen bee is kept below the upper boxes in the hive, called supers, by a wire or plastic grid that the queen is too large to fit through. This is called the queen excluder. Because the bees can't raise brood above the excluder, only honey is stored in the supers. As the season progresses, the bee-keeper adds more supers to the hive until it is time to harvest the honey. A special one-way valve is fitted in place of the queen excluder and gradually all the bees are forced into the lowest part of the hive. It takes up to 48 hours for the bees to clear from the supers. The bee-keeper can then simply lift off the super boxes containing honeycomb. The honey is extracted from the comb using centrifugal force in a machine called a spinner, which looks like an old-fashioned spin dryer. The bees don't really miss the honey, as a strong colony can produce two to three times more honey than they need. If necessary, the bee-keeper will feed sugar syrup to the bees in the autumn to compensate for the loss of honey.

QUALITY, NOT QUANTITY

The reason that a small-scale producer can usually supply superior quality honey is down to freshness. In addition to sugars, honey is a complex blend of many trace substances, some of which are volatile and diminish quickly after the bees have produced it. These are typically the elements that contribute to the subtle taste and pleasant floral aromatic qualities. They are also the ones easily lost in the mass-produced product. To obtain a consistent long-life product the mass producer needs to flash heat-treat and mechanically thrash the honey. A blend is then produced from several, often geographically remote, sources. The result is a consistent but some would say bland honey that could take two years or more from bee to toast.

FILTERING

Leaving the freshly extracted honey for 24 hours before filtering is beneficial, especially if stored in a warming cabinet. The honey will be thinner and most debris will have floated to the surface, making filtering a fast, easy operation. Warmed honey filters much more easily than cold honey so it is warmed a little to 35–40°C (95–104°F) for a few days. Any longer and a by-product of the honey degrading called HMF (Hydroxy Methyl Furfuraldehyde) starts to rise. This is not harmful but can be used by authorities as an indicator of abused or adulterated honey. The hotter the honey gets, the faster this breakdown happens. Prolonged temperatures in excess of 35°C (95°F) will also cause an undesirable change in flavour. It is best to use two or three filters cascaded together, for example two kitchen sieves, coarse then fine, and finally a nylon or scrim filter cloth. The honey should flow from a large container fitted with a honey tap through the filters and into an equally large container.

STORAGE

Honey absorbs water, so it should be stored in clean, plastic food grade containers with air-tight lids. When pre-packed for retail sale in quantities of more than 50 g honey can only legally be packed in the following net weights: 57 g (⅛ lb), 113 g (¼ lb), 227 g (½ lb), 340 g (¾ lb), 454 g (1 lb), 680 g (1½ lb) or multiples of 454 g. Honey of less than 50 g, chunk honey and comb honey may be packed in any weight.

YIELDS

This can range from nothing to about 27 kg (60 lb) in a good season, but typically 13–23 kg (30–50 lb per hive). It could be worse than nothing, as you may need to feed your bees to keep them alive in a bad year!

CAUTION: OIL SEED RAPE

I've never liked the stuff that seems to have taken over vast tracts of the countryside. When I was a primary teacher, I remember one year having to take the children off the school field during the flowering season, as several pupils with asthma were finding it difficult to breathe. Because our field backed on to a field of OSR, a colleague had trouble with her asthma every time she taught PE outside. Eventually the problem diminished, when the farmer was not allowed to grow it next to the school any more, but whenever I drive past a field of OSR I have to close the windows. The smell, if you haven't had the pleasure, is sweet, sickly and lingering, and the colour is a violent, acid yellow.

I didn't know until I visited Graham's site that OSR also causes immense problems for bee-keepers. OSR (in the USA, known as Canola) honey granulates into a solid very quickly and it must be extracted before it sets in the comb. OSR is now planted in the late autumn (winter rape) to start flowering in the spring as early as March. It can also be planted in the spring (spring rape) to flower later, maybe as late as July or August. This prolonged season can make it a real nuisance, as bees first work on winter OSR and then go on to spring OSR. It then dominates the honey crop for all that season, as the bees prefer OSR nectar to almost all other potential nectar sources.

If you leave it until the honey is fully capped, as is good advice for all other honeys, then you're too late. Instead the bees should have started to cap (seal it with a thin layer of wax) some of the honey on the frame. Otherwise you end up with solid honey stuck fast in the comb.

DISEASE

This is a malaise that has been spreading through the nation's bee colonies with alarming implications because of foreign diseases and the spread of drug resistance among infectious bees. There has been a serious decline in the bee population and the implications, not only for honey production but also for other agricultural industries, are immense. To restore populations bees have been imported from Europe and Australia, although it is unclear if this will be a long-term solution. The crisis can be traced back to the nineties when hives were first struck by *varroa destructor*. This parasitic mite feeds off the bodily fluids of bees, resulting in plummeting populations among wild swarms, which have virtually been eradicated. The only colonies surviving are tended by keepers. Without a keeper to help, the feral bees only survive for a short time because of the disease. A relaxing of rules which allows people to import bees from other countries has only increased the risk of new disease entering Britain. Parasites, like the American Fowl Brood and the Small Hive Beetle, infect other countries' bees, and their arrival in Britain is now inevitable. A lot of keepers and farmers in Britain who have contracts with orchard owners, to provide pollination of their trees, are now having to import them.

However, only single queen bees are brought into the country, which limits the prospects for the spread of infections. Packages of queen bees arrive along with workers to provide her with food, but the workers are destroyed, leaving only the queen, who is gradually introduced to a new hive, where she is eventually accepted.

BEE-KEEPING AS A HOBBY

Bee-keeping is a seasonal hobby, although there are a number of routine jobs to carry out.

MONTHLY TASKS

Jan	Check roofs and entrances for blockages by leaves or snow.
Feb	Check hives for food, feed as necessary.
Mar	Change/clean floor. Continue to monitor food levels. Monitor Varroa levels, this continues through the season from now on. High levels of mites found will need treating sooner rather than later.
April	First inspection on mild day, checking health, food, queen is ok (queenright). Replace old comb
May	Start weekly swarm prevention inspections. Add supers (honey boxes) as necessary. Start to breed new queens as part of your swarm prevention and good management.
June	Continue weekly swarm prevention inspections and add supers. If the bees have been getting nectar from early oil seed rape then this honey will need to be removed by now.
July	Keep adding supers and inspecting for swarming.
Aug	Remove main honey crop. Best time to treat for Varroa by using Varroacides. Restrict the entrance to prevent other bees or wasps from robbing your hives.
Sept	Feed for the winter. Sort out how many hives you want to start next year with by reducing your hive count, combining two into one.
Oct	No further internal inspections from now on. Fit mouse guards for the onset of winter.
Nov	Check externals routinely, especially after severe weather, in case of storm damage.
Dec	As October but you should be attending your local association meetings and making your plans for next year based on this year's experiences.

Types
of Honey

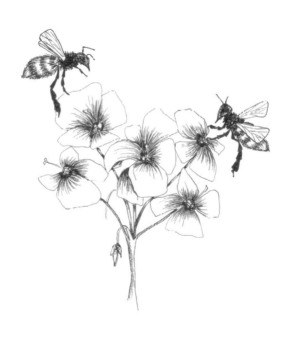

Honey exists in various forms and there are a number of processes to which it may be subjected.

MONOFLORAL HONEY
When bees have access to large areas of one kind of flower, such as clover, basswood, heather, goldenrod, or buckwheat, they produce honey with a flavour and colour typical of that particular plant. These monofloral honeys are not as commonly produced as blends. Most honeys available in shops and outlets are produced from a variety of different sources and are a blend of flower types. Many of the monoflorals, such as manuka, nodding thistle or honeydew, come from New Zealand.

BRITISH MONOFLORAL HONEY
These tend to focus on heather and sea lavender. Obviously the commercial production of heather honey coincides with the upland and moorland regions, where heather dominates the landscape. These are found in the Lake District, Dartmoor, Exmoor and the Quantocks, the Peak District and the Yorkshire Moors. Sea lavender is produced along the coastal areas of East Anglia and in Scotland.

HEATHER HONEY
Production of heather honey involves moving the bees up to the moors between May and July, to forage on the flowering heathers. Bee-keepers are concerned about the proximity of oil seed rape plants, which will contaminate the honey and cause it to crystallise quickly, setting solid in the combs. Nectar and pollen from heathers, mainly ling and bell heather, create honey with a strong taste and dark colour. The benefits to the landscape of managed heather moorlands are also best for honey production. Management includes the periodic burning of heather to encourage young growth, leading to increased productivity for bees.

It is interesting to note that Dartmoor honey was recorded in the *Domesday Book*. One of the main producers is Buckfast Abbey, where a strain of bee has been produced from a cross between the native English bee and the Italian bee. This strain is disinclined to swarm and has excellent honey-gathering abilities.

Towards the end of July the hives are taken up to the Dartmoor heather for the flowering season from August to early September. Afterwards the bees are returned to the Abbey, an operation which takes about ten days.

SEA LAVENDER HONEY
This honey is pale yellow to green when runny, but crystallises quickly to a smooth texture with a mild but distinct flavour. Sea lavender, a member of the statice family, often grown for drying, grows on the mudflats of the tidal salt marshes around the Thames estuary, the Norfolk and Suffolk coastlines and the coast of Scotland. These are areas where erosion by the sea has always been a problem, and a system of dykes, sea walls and channels has been applied to control the water. This has created a perfect habitat for sea lavender and the honey can be collected in good quantities. Most of this honey is consumed locally, obviously by people who appreciate it. Hives are moved to the flowering areas along the river channels in August. This is a time when the flowering season of most other sources is nearly over, so it is a welcome source of nectar.

APPLE BLOSSOM HONEY
This is produced in Devon and in the orchards of Kent, the Garden of England. Most other monofloral honeys are not produced on a commercial basis in the UK and are only available in limited quantities from local producers.

NAMED HONEYS
Named honeys from other parts of the world tend to be derived from a mixture of flowers with the name of the honey being the dominant species of flower. Examples in the USA would be orange blossom, tupelo and sourwood, although there are monofloral varieties of these as well. In France, lavender and acacia seem to be prevalent and in Greece wild thyme honey is very popular.

ORGANIC HONEY
Organic honey is almost impossible to produce commercially in Europe because the flying range of bees 3 miles (4.8 km) will nearly always be within reach of conventional agriculture, where chemicals will have been

used in one way or another. There are, however, some organic honeys produced on a small scale, especially on islands such as the Scottish Isles.

Like many good wines produced in Europe, honey flavour and colour can vary from year to year, depending on weather in the case of wines and also on the prevalent species of plants with honey. Honey is rich in antioxidants and antibacterial qualities, although some are considered to be healthier than others. The lingering flavours, giving an indication of their derivation, make different honeys perfect for different uses. There are more than 300 floral sources for honey in the USA, each with a distinct colour and flavour. Colours range from virtually colourless to dark brown, and flavours from mild to bitter. As a general rule, the lighter the honey the milder the taste. Below is a quick summary of the aroma, flavour and characteristics of numerous monofloral honeys from around the world. This list is not exhaustive and I don't claim to have tasted them all. Being diabetic, I have to limit my intake of honey, unfortunately.

NAME	CHARACTERISTICS	AROMA
Acacia	Clear, light to colourless. Remains liquified for long periods; good with ricotta cheese	vanilla and floral
Alfalfa	High in dextrose, granulates quickly	beeswax
Avocado	Smooth, velvety, brown sugar or molasses	flowery
Blackberry	Thick, viscous appearance, but transparent	flowery perfume
Blueberry	Runny, delicate	lemony, unripened fruit
Buckwheat	Dark, sharp with a lingering aftertaste of molasses	pungent
Chestnut	Dark amber, remains liquified for a long time. Very high in minerals	intense, pungent
Clover	Clear, light and yellowy, good table honey	sweet and slightly spicy
Cranberry	Mild and fruity	fruity

Eucalyptus	Dark amber to grey, good with cheese and herbal teas	sweet, clovery
Galberry	Dark and thick	very flowery
Golden rod	Unripe honey has putrid smell, used by bakeries	distinctive
Heather	Towards orange in colour. Doesn't cloud herbal teas	fresh and flowery
Honeydew*	Dense, dark, remains liquified, rich in mineral salts	sweet
Lavender	Light and creamy	flowery
Leatherwood	Generally considered too strong in unblended form	spicy
Lime tree	Clear, good for herbal teas	strong perfume
Manuka	Renowned for bacterial healing qualities	earthy
Mesquite	Produced from sweet-smoky-smelling tree	smoky
Nodding thistle	Light coloured, mild	flowery perfume
Orange blossom	Crystallises to a consistent, white colour	orange blossom, citrus
Rata	Very white in colour	mild
Sage	Thick and viscous, doesn't granulate	sweet, unripe fruit
Sourwood	Astringent, anise	liquorice
Soybean	Dark, thick with fruity aftertaste	sharp and strong
Star thistle	Light colour, thick	spicy, anise
Strawberry tree	Very rare Italian, clear amber to grey	pungent
Sunflower	Yellow, crystallises rapidly, used in biscuits and nougat	fruity, low aroma
Tawari	Best when young	subtle, mild
Thyme	Burnt grass colour; high in antibacterial qualities	intense
Tupelo	Light amber with greenish cast from Florida	herbal
Viper's bugloss	Chewy texture; keep in fridge as chewy snack	flowery

*Honeydew honey is different from other honeys in that it is produced from forest zones where aphids exude sugary secretion after sucking sap from the leaves and surfaces of plants.

POLYFLORAL HONEY
Bees also make natural blends of honey from many different flowers, in areas where no one flower predominates. This is known as polyfloral honey. Honeys are also blended by commercial producers during packing to produce a consistent taste combination that can be replicated, time after time.

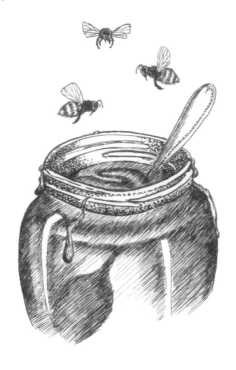

HONEY GLOSSARY

HONEY
COMB HONEY Honey-filled beeswax comb as stored directly by the bees.
CHUNK HONEY Comb honey in a jar with liquid honey poured around it.
BLENDED HONEY A mixture of two or more honeys differing in floral source, colour, flavour, density or geographic origin.
CRYSTALLISED or *GRANULATED HONEY* Honey in which part of the natural glucose content has spontaneously crystallised. Granulated honey is made by blending one part finely granulated honey with nine parts liquid honey.

The mixture is stored at about 14°C (57°F) until it becomes firm. To reliquify naturally granulated honey, put the container in a double boiler or water bath at about 63°C (145°F). Loosen or remove the container lid and stir the honey once or twice while it is heating. As soon as the granules are dissolved, remove the honey from the heat and let it cool quickly. Honey that is partially granulated is not going bad.

FILTERED HONEY Honey processed by filtration to remove pollen grains and extraneous solids.

LIQUID HONEY Prepared by cutting off the wax cappings and whirling the comb in a honey extractor, where centrifugal force moves the honey out of the cells.

RAW HONEY Honey as it exists in the beehive or as obtained by extraction, settling or straining. No heating takes place.

STRAINED HONEY Honey which has been passed through a mesh to remove pieces of wax, propolis or other matter, without removing pollen.

WHIPPED, CHURNED or *CREAMED HONEY* Honey processed, by controlled *crystallisation*, to a smooth, spreadable consistency. This is popular in the USA and is also called candied honey or honey fondant.

BEESWAX

Wax is produced by the youngest bees, from 12 to 18 days old, that cluster together in large numbers to raise their body temperature. After they have consumed copious amounts of honey, they slowly excrete, through wax-producing glands under their abdomen, slivers of wax about the size of a pinhead. Other worker bees massage

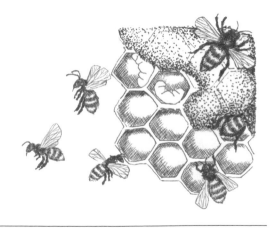

the harvested wax scales and take them to use in cell construction or to cap cells containing honey in other parts of the hive. To produce a pound of wax, bees use about 2.7 kg (6 lb) of honey. They normally stop making wax just after the summer solstice.

Although modern scientific processes have developed a number of other substances to meet the wax needs of today, many craftsmen still prefer the unique qualities of beeswax, a mixture that cannot be duplicated artificially. Its value as a commodity has been treasured by most world cultures, and beeswax has always commanded a high price. It enjoys use in candle making, batik designs, cosmetic products and in the making and upkeep of musical instruments and furniture.

ROYAL JELLY

This is the food fed to a potential queen larva. It is creamy white and very rich in protein and fatty acids. It is produced by the mouth glands of worker bees and used to feed developing young. All bee larvae are fed royal jelly for the first three days of development. Queen larvae are fed it during their entire larval development. Each queen needs only a teaspoon of royal jelly. As a health product, it is very expensive and almost tasteless. Only small quantities can be removed from the hives.

PROPOLIS

This is a resin collected by the bees from trees and plants. When taken back to the hive it is mixed with wax and used for a variety of protective as well as defensive purposes. Propolis has antibacterial, antifungal and anti-inflammatory properties and has been used by man for over 3,000 years.

The resin is made of about 50% resin, 30% wax, 10% essential oils and 5% pollen. Propolis is used by the bees as a sticky filler and glue to protect the hive as a sterile environment. Over the last 30 years medical research has begun to uncover the secrets of propolis as a natural antibiotic. The substance can now be bought as a tincture to treat many ailments.

The Health Benefits of Using Honey

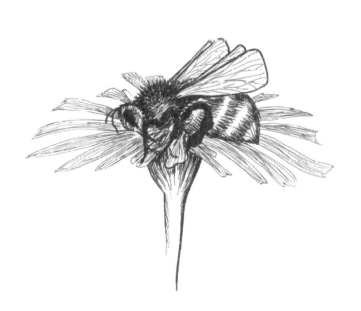

Honey has been used to promote healing for centuries. Ancient civilisations knew about its therapeutic value as well as its sweetening value and probably revered honey precisely because it made people feel better. Who didn't have honey and lemon drinks given for a sore throat or cough as a child? Just look at the range of home remedies using honey with other renowned natural products and foodstuffs, including vinegar and porridge, or read my other books! Honey is chemically compatible with a wide variety of products. Its pH is in a range common to many foods.

Nutritionally, natural honey contains about 75–80% sugar and the rest is a mixture of water, minerals including phosphorus, calcium and magnesium, and enzymes. Honey is high in energy. One teaspoon of honey gives about 15 calories, but because it is a natural product the composition of honey is highly variable.

A typical blended honey contains the following, per 100 g:

Energy	307 calories
Protein	0.4 g
Carbohydrates (all sugar)	76.4 g
Sodium	trace
Fat	nil

A monofloral, unpasteurised honey may contain, per 100 g:

Total sugars	77.9 g
Of which	
Fructose	38.2 g
Glucose	31.0 g
Sucrose	1.5 g
Maltose	7.2 g
Water	17.1 g
Other carbohydrates	4.2 g
Minerals, vitamins	
& enzymes	0.5 g

Minerals may include traces of calcium, iron, zinc, potassium, magnesium, selenium and manganese. There may be traces of vitamin B (riboflavin, niacin) and a small amount of vitamin C.

YOU GET IT FROM THE BEES — NOT YOUR GP!
Modern science has allowed us to look more carefully at the claims of antibacterial properties and at the composition of honey. Research has suggested that the reason honey prevents microbes growing may be because:

- It is low in water activity
- Its viscosity limits the dissolving of oxygen
- It has a high carbon to nitrogen ratio
- The formation of hydrogen peroxide through chemical change prevents growth of bacteria such as E.coli
- It lacks protein and has a high sugar content
- It has a low pH value
- It has the benefits of phytochemicals (plant chemicals with antibacterial properties) which are influenced by bee enzymes

It has also been suggested that darker honeys and those with high water content have the potential to be stronger in their antioxidant properties.

Honey has inherent properties that discourage the growth or persistence of many micro-organisms. The microbes that may be found in honey are mostly yeasts and spore-forming bacteria. No vegetative forms of bacterial spores have been found in honey.

THE ALCHEMY OF THE HONEY BEE & OTHER SCIENTIFIC FACTS

YEASTS
All natural honeys contain sugar-tolerant yeasts. They are destroyed by pasteurisation.

FERMENTATION
This will not occur in honey that has carbohydrate content greater than 83%, moisture content less than 17.1%, a storage temperature less than 52°F (11°C) or that has been heat-treated. The process of warming honey prior to filtration also acts to purify it but not pasteurise it. If properly extracted, treated and stored, honey should not ferment.

FREEZING POINT

The freezing point of a 15% honey solution is about −1.45°C (29°F). A 68% honey solution freezes at −5.8°C (22°F).

PASTEURISATION

Some honey is heat-treated to prevent unwanted fermentation and to delay crystallisation. One common heat treatment is 77°C (170°F) for two minutes followed by rapid cooling to 54°C (130°F). Honey may be damaged by too much heat.

ENZYMES

The enzymes present in honey aid in the digestion of raw sugars and starch. The sugar content in honey is in a very simple, predigested form, directly absorbed by our body. Normal sugar has to be broken down into simpler forms to be digested and absorbed. Honey may aid digestion, but as the calorific content is high, it won't keep you slim. Be aware also that honey, like other sugary food, rots your teeth.

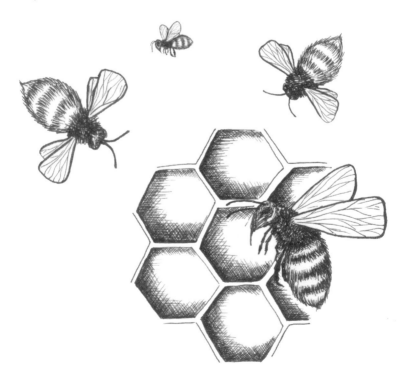

HEAL ME, HONEY!
USES FOR HEALTH AND PERSONAL CARE

NOT FOR YOU, BABY
Special mention should be made on the subject of giving honey to infants under one year of age. Infant botulism is a rare but serious paralytic disease caused by a micro-organism. Spores can germinate, grow and produce toxin in the lower bowel of some infants. Honey is a potential source of these spores and infants are susceptible until their intestinal bacteria develop. Older children and adults are normally able to ingest the spores without harm.

DIABETES AND HONEY
Honey may be included in a diabetic diet, but diabetics must comply with the medical regime and diet instructions prescribed by their individual healthcare providers, to keep blood sugar levels under control.
As always, there are pros and cons. The answer for the control of my own diabetes, type 2, is to maintain a balance and limit the use of honey, along with sugar, salt, sugar substitutes, red meats, fats, etc., while eating plenty of fresh fruit and vegetables, fish, white meat and whole grain cereals like oats. Honey is a natural product and has many other benefits to offer, so I think it worth including in my diet, in moderation.

The following suggestions are passed on as possible solutions to a range of minor ailments, or as preventative suggestions for more serious conditions. You should always seek medical advice if in doubt, or are taking prescribed medicines already. Many of these are from obscure sources with unproven scientific results, so should be taken with a pinch of salt . . . or honey.

ARTHRITIS
As a topical application:
Take one tablespoon of honey to two tablespoons of lukewarm water. Add a small teaspoon of cinnamon powder, make a paste and massage it onto the affected part of the body.

As a honey and cinnamon drink:
Take one cup of hot water with two dessertspoons of honey and a small teaspoon of cinnamon powder three times a day.

Vinegar drink:
Drink a glass of water with two teaspoons of cider vinegar and two teaspoons of honey three times a day. It dissolves the crystal deposits of uric acid that form between joints.

Danish remedy:
Take one tablespoon of honey and half a teaspoon of cinnamon powder before breakfast.

While this seems to be effective, always ask your doctor before attempting to diagnose yourself or deciding upon medication to alleviate any symptoms.

BAD BREATH
Some people in South America gargle with one teaspoon of honey and cinnamon powder mixed in hot water every morning, so that their breath stays fresh throughout the day.

BOILS
Boils are quite painful and at times have to be lanced. One tablespoon of cider vinegar and one tablespoon of honey mixed in a cup of hot water at least twice a day may bring relief; you should also drink plenty of water. If the boil does come to a head where it is going to open, continue to drink the vinegar and honey tea and the water. Use hot packs on the boil for 15 to 20 minutes three times a day. What is also important is not to squeeze a boil.

BLADDER INFECTIONS
Take two tablespoons of cinnamon powder and one teaspoon of honey in a glass of lukewarm water.

CHOLESTEROL
Apparently, two tablespoons of honey and three teaspoons of cinnamon mixed in water reduced the level of cholesterol in the blood by 10% within two hours in one experiment.

Instead of jam, make a paste of honey and cinnamon powder. Spread on bread or toast. This is said to reduce the cholesterol from eating buttered, jammy equivalents.

COLITIS
Cider vinegar and honey have been used effectively in the treatment of colitis. Take two teaspoons of cider vinegar and honey with water, three times a day.

CONSTIPATION
As far as constipation is concerned, honey is, apparently, a popular laxative.

COUGHS
There are many types of coughs, and these should be treated with reference to their nature and intensity. However, the vinegar and honey treatment may help some types.

Tickly cough:
Two teaspoons of cider vinegar and two of honey mixed with a glassful of water should be taken before meals, or when the irritation occurs. In the evening it would be an idea to have this mixture by your bed so that it can be sipped during the night.

If you are really brave, or desperate, try this one:
Relieve a cough by mixing half a cup of apple cider vinegar, half a cup of water, one teaspoon of cayenne pepper, and four teaspoons of honey. Take a tablespoon when the cough starts and another tablespoon at bedtime.

DETOX AND ENERGISER
Taking honey with hot water and a slice of lemon is a great way to kick-start your day. It provides an energy boost that is much better for you than caffeine.

ECZEMA
Take cider vinegar and honey in a glassful of water three times a day, with meals. Under no circumstances should salt be taken, as this can aggravate the eczema condition considerably.

EYES — TIRED AND SORE

The cider vinegar therapy together with honey are the essential ingredients here. Take two teaspoons of each in a glassful of water, three times a day. This mixture delays the onset of tired and sore eyes which are usually apparent in later life, as it supplies them with those vital elements essential to their health and function.

FATIGUE

Chronic fatigue is a warning that the body needs some attention. To remedy a poor quality sleep, honey is highly recommended, as it acts as a sedative to the body. Twenty minutes after the honey has been taken into the mouth it has been digested and absorbed into the body. This is because it is a predigested sugar, already digested in the stomach of the honey bee, and it requires no effort on the part of the human stomach to digest. Keep the following mixture by your bedside, to be taken as indicated: three teaspoons of apple cider vinegar to 275 ml (½ pint) of honey.

Take two teaspoons of the mixture before retiring. This should induce sound sleep within an hour. If, however, you have been unable to sleep within this period, repeat the dosage.

Senior citizens who take honey and cinnamon powder in equal parts, are more alert and flexible. Half a tablespoon of honey taken in a glass of water and sprinkled with cinnamon powder should be taken in the afternoon at about 3 p.m. when the vitality of the body starts to decrease.

FLATULENCE

According to studies done in India and Japan, if honey is taken with cinnamon powder the stomach is relieved of gas.

HAIR LOSS

Apply a paste of warm olive oil, one tablespoon of honey and one teaspoon of cinnamon powder before a bath. Keep it on for about 15 minutes before washing the hair.

HAY FEVER

I've seen amazing results based on this idea, admittedly only in one patient, but I was impressed by the theory of oral tolerance, which reasons that humans become accustomed to things they ingest. If people eat local pollens via pollen-rich honey, allergic pollen reaction like hay fever in the spring and summer should diminish. Although it sounds strange it worked for my daughter's boyfriend without him having to take medication. Obviously, you have to know which pollens you are allergic to for it to work properly.

This ailment is marked by watery eyes, sneezing and running nose, in other words there is an excess of fluid which the body is drastically trying to offload. For another effective relief use honey and cider vinegar. Take a tablespoonful of honey after each meal for approximately a fortnight before the onset of the hay-fever season. Two teaspoons of cider vinegar and two of honey in a glass of water, three times a day, should then be taken. This dosage should be maintained during the entire hay-fever season.

HEADACHES

Many people have had relief from headaches by the use of honey. Two teaspoons taken at each meal may well prevent an attack.

HEALING PROPERTIES

Several factors may account for honey's healing properties. Bacterial infections require water to thrive, but the sugars in honey attract water, so may deprive bacteria. Bee pollen and propolis enzymes are present in honey. These work from within the honey to sterilise wounds and assist healing. Glucose oxidase found in honey combines with water and produces hydrogen peroxide, of which the antiseptic properties are released when honey touches the skin. Various types of honey contain different antibacterial substances.

HIGH BLOOD PRESSURE

Emphasis for sufferers is on the natural — foods that are given in the form of fresh fruits, vegetables and honey —

rather than high protein foods which include eggs, meat, milk, cheese, nuts, beans, etc. A balance must be maintained between proteins and carbohydrates. The following dosage should be taken: two teaspoons of apple cider vinegar and honey in a glass of water — up to three or four times a day.

IMMUNE SYSTEM
Daily use of honey strengthens the immune system and protects the body from bacteria and viral attacks. Honey contains various vitamins and iron. Constant use of honey strengthens the white blood corpuscles to fight bacteria and viral diseases.

INDIGESTION
Cinnamon powder, sprinkled on two tablespoons of honey taken before food, relieves acidity and aids digestion. It could also make you put on a lot of weight.

INFERTILITY IN MEN
If impotent men regularly take two tablespoons of honey before going to sleep, their problem will apparently be solved.

INFERTILITY IN WOMEN
In the Far East, women who cannot conceive take a pinch of cinnamon powder in half a teaspoon of honey and apply it to the gums frequently throughout the day, so that it slowly mixes with the saliva and enters the body.

IMPOTENCE, PREMATURE EJACULATION AND VIRILITY
Powdered cardamom seeds boiled with milk and mixed in a glass with a spoon of honey is believed to be an excellent remedy against impotence and premature ejaculation, and promotes virility.

In the East, ginger has lived up to its reputation of being a powerful herb. Indian literature recommends a mixture of ginger juice, honey and half-boiled eggs, taken nightly for a month, as a remedy against impotence.

INSOMNIA

There have been excellent results with the cider vinegar and honey treatment as follows: two teaspoons of cider vinegar and two of honey in a glass of water to be taken before retiring. It would also be beneficial to have a glass of this mixture by the bedside to sip if needed.

LONGEVITY

Tea made with honey and cinnamon arrests the ravages of old age, when taken regularly. Take four teaspoons of honey, one teaspoon of cinnamon powder and three cups of water and boil to make a tea. Drink during the course of the day. It keeps the skin fresh and soft and is said to slow down the onset of old age. Another suggestion is to mix honey, cornflour and limejuice. This acts as a good moisturiser and helps dry skin problems. See the section on beauty treatments for more ideas.

MOUTH INFECTIONS

Despite rotting teeth, honey has active antibiotic properties and disinfects the mouth.

PIMPLES

Mix three tablespoons of honey and one teaspoon of cinnamon powder. Apply this paste on the pimples before sleeping and wash it off next morning with warm water. Repeat daily for two weeks.

PREVENTION OF SCARRING

When honey is exposed to air, it draws in moisture. This may help to prevent scarring by keeping skin moist and helping in the growth of new skin. Additionally, it helps to stop dressings becoming stuck to an open wound. For these reasons honey can be used as a moisturiser and skin care product. See page 69.

SEDATIVE

Two tablespoons of honey in a glass of hot milk is said to be a good sedative.

SORE THROAT

A gargle made from apple cider vinegar and water could prove to be a great relief for a sore throat — be that a bacterial or virus infection. Use a 50/50 mixture, and spit out the solution after gargling, which should be repeated every hour. After gargling rinse the mouth with clean water to prevent the acid from eroding the enamel on your teeth. Honey is good for sore throats, coughs and colds. Honey and lemon juice in equal parts, dissolved in hot water, is a soothing drink.

THIRST QUENCHER
In addition to its excellent medicinal properties, honey is supposed to be a good thirst quencher. Nomadic travellers take honey and water across deserts, and honey has been used to sweeten tea and coffee for centuries.

TOOTHACHE
Since honey is a sugar and sugar rots teeth, this remedy sounds like pouring petrol on the flames.

Make a paste of one teaspoon of cinnamon powder and five teaspoons of honey. Apply to the aching tooth three times a day. Better still, visit your dentist regularly!

ULCERS
Honey helps in the healing and sterilising of wounds and ulcers and helps the growth of new skin. Manuka honey is especially important, as it is effective against more resistant bacteria. It is this type of honey that has been shown to be very good in treating some stomach ulcers and sore throats.

WEIGHT LOSS
Combine one tablespoon of apple cider vinegar and one tablespoon of honey in a 227 ml (8 oz) glass of unsweetened grapefruit juice. Drink one glass before each meal as an appetite suppressant. An alternative suggestion is to drink honey and cinnamon powder boiled in a cup of water, before breakfast and at night before sleeping.

BEE VENOM THERAPY

Many people in the Far East and Eastern Europe advocate this drastic therapy to treat rheumatic diseases, arthritis, multiple sclerosis and a host of other ailments. It should, however, only be used after careful thought and discussion with an apitherapist and a doctor. The therapy should be carefully monitored: you don't just annoy a bee until it stings you. Enthusiasts recommend using all hive products which work together to strengthen your immune system. This means using royal jelly, propolis, pollen capsules, along with raw, unprocessed honey, St John's wort, ginkgo, ginseng, garlic and vitamin C daily.

REACTION TO BEE VENOM

Bee venom is the product of the bee's sting and some people are allergic to it. There are many reactions that can happen, but normally the stings provoke a localised reaction, with redness and swelling surrounding the sting area. A more severe reaction will result when the swelling increases to the whole limb, causing problems with movement.

The most severe reactions occur when the person stung has intensive skin redness, irritation and difficulty in breathing, possibly resulting in loss of consciousness. This is also known as anaphylactic reaction and requires urgent medical help.

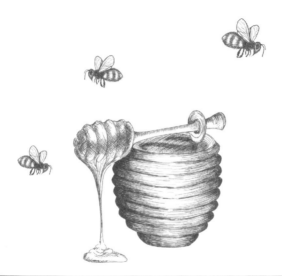

Beauty Treatments with Honey

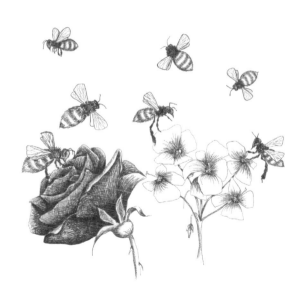

Cleopatra knew a thing or two about beauty. Her fabled baths of milk and honey worked because honey is a humectant, which means it attracts and retains moisture. (This is also why it is so useful in baking.)

You might like to try some of these ideas for beauty treatments. If you have sensitive skin, try any new product, natural or otherwise, on a small area of skin first, then wait for a while to see if there is any adverse reaction. Also be aware that, when using oats with honey and oils, you can block drains, so do the environmentally friendly thing and remove face packs and cleansers with care. Don't mix metric and imperial quantities within a recipe, as there will be small discrepancies between equivalent weights.

Some of the ideas are really simple, involving only everyday ingredients from the store cupboard, some are a little more indulgent and some are just whacky!

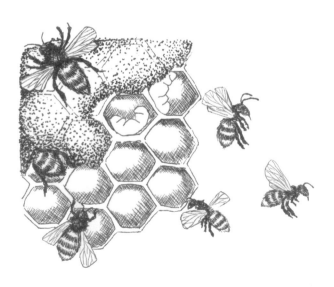

BEAUTY TREATMENT RECIPES

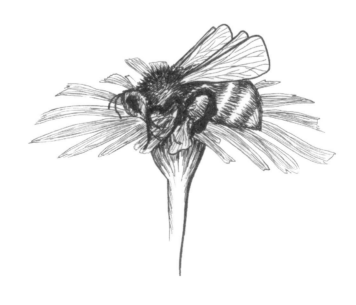

A VERY SIMPLE MOISTURE MASK, CLEOPATRA-STYLE

You will need:

2 tablespoons honey

2 teaspoons milk

Method:

Mix the honey with milk. Smooth over the face and throat. Leave for 10 minutes before rinsing off with warm water.

FIRMING FACE MASK

You will need:

1 tablespoon honey

1 egg white

1 teaspoon glycerine

approx. 2 tablespoons cornflour

Method:

Whisk together all ingredients and enough cornflour to form a paste. Smooth over the face and throat. Leave on for 10 minutes while you relax, before rinsing off with lukewarm water.

HONEY AND ALMOND SCRUB

You will need:

8 whole, unblanched almonds

2 tablespoons rolled oats

1 tablespoon honey

2 teaspoons yoghurt

Method:

Put the almonds and oats into a blender and grind until fine. Mix with the honey and yoghurt. Apply to the face and neck, avoiding the eyes, and leave for up to 10 minutes. Massage with wet hands to gently exfoliate. Rinse off and pat dry.

HAWAIIAN FACIAL

You will need: for 2 treatments

   ½ ripe papaya
   ½ cup fresh pineapple, diced
   2 tablespoons green tea
   2 tablespoons honey

Method:
Using green tea bags would make this simpler but, if not,
infuse the green tea in less than half a cup of boiling
water. While this is cooling, peel the papaya and remove
the seeds. Blend the papaya and pineapple until puréed.
Combine the honey with the fruit and add the cooled
green tea (don't make it too runny). Mix well. Apply to
the face with your finger tips and rest for 10 to 15
minutes. Remove completely with tepid water and
tissues. Store the surplus in a covered container in the
fridge for up to a week.

HONEY, ALMOND AND LEMON CLEANSER

You will need:

   1 tablespoon honey
   2 tablespoons finely ground almonds
   ½ teaspoon lemon juice

Method:
Mix all the ingredients and dab gently on to the face.
Rinse off with warm water.

CUCUMBER AND HONEY EYE NOURISHER

Always be careful when applying new ingredients to the
face, especially on the delicate skin under the eyes.
Avoid getting any of the ingredients into your eyes.
This recipe should reduce puffiness, and cool and refresh
the contour under the eyes.

You will need:

½ tablespoon aloe vera gel
1 teaspoon cucumber, peeled with seeds removed
½ teaspoon honey
½ teaspoon camomile tea

Method:
Infuse the camomile tea in a small amount of boiling water (about an eggcupful). While this cools blend the cucumber, aloe vera and honey. Add the cooled camomile tea and mix thoroughly. Chill the cream before applying gently under the eyes. Store the surplus in a covered dish in the fridge for up to a week.

AVOCADO AND CUCUMBER FACE MASK

You will need:

¼ of a cucumber, peeled and chopped
½ an avocado
3 tablespoons finely powdered oats
3 tablespoons of water
1 tablespoon fresh lemon juice
1 teaspoon honey
8–9 tablespoons green clay or kaolin
Few drops of essential oils (optional)

Method:
Purée the cucumber and avocado flesh in a food processor with water and lemon juice until smooth. Add the oats, honey and essential oils. Pour the mix into a bowl and then whisk in the clay. Apply to the face and neck and leave on for 20 to 30 minutes. Rinse off with warm water, then use a toner and moisturiser.

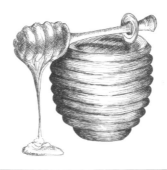

PUMPKIN FACE MASK

Pumpkins are full of betacarotene and vitamin A, making them especially nourishing for your skin. This sounds an ideal recipe to try at Halloween time. You might not even need a mask!

You will need:
- 1 miniature pumpkin, or portion of a larger one
- 4 pineapple chunks
- 1 tablespoon finely powdered oats
- 1 tablespoon finely powdered almonds
- 1 teaspoon milk
- 1 teaspoon honey
- 1 teaspoon olive oil
- 2 drops rose geranium essential oil

Method:
Use a sharp knife to core the pumpkin and slice on a cutting board. Cut about 6 to 8 pieces. Place pumpkin pieces (including seeds) in a microwave-safe dish with about ¼ cup of water. Microwave for about 2 minutes until the flesh is soft. Allow to cool. Cut the peel off. Place the pumpkin flesh, seeds and strings into a small food processor with the pineapple and blend until smooth. Add oats, almonds, milk and honey in that order, processing after each addition. Add the oil, essential oil and stir. The texture should be rich and smooth, with just a slight graininess from the almonds.

To use, apply to cleaned and toned face and neck skin. Rest for 15 minutes. Rinse well with warm water and follow with moisturiser.

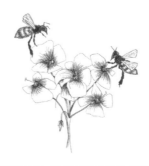

BANANA BALM

This is a cleanser and moisturiser in one and suits all skin types, especially dry. The essential oil is optional.

You will need:
½ fresh banana
1 tablespoon fresh whipping cream, lightly warmed
1 teaspoon honey, slightly warmed
Approximately 1 tablespoon fine oatmeal
Few drops essential oil (optional)

Method:
Mash the banana to a creamy pulp. Warm the honey and whipping cream in a microwave for about 15 seconds. Stir well, then add to the banana pulp.
Add the oats and essential oil and stir again.
To use, massage over dampened skin using gentle, sweeping, upward motions. Rinse well and follow with a toner and moisturiser.

CUCUMBER FACE MASK FOR SENSITIVE SKIN

You will need:
¼ large cucumber, peeled and seeded
1 tablespoon whipping cream
½ tablespoon clear honey
About 8 teaspoons finely powdered oats

Method:
Place the peeled and seeded cucumber in a blender and process until liquified. Add the whipping cream and honey and process until smooth. Add the oats and process further until a paste-like mixture is formed. (Add more oats if the cucumber is very watery.) Smooth a thick layer over clean skin and rest for 15 minutes. Rinse with warm water and apply moisturiser.

DEEP FACIAL HONEY AND OATMEAL CLEANSER

You will need:
 1 tablespoon honey
 1 tablespoon oatmeal
 2 slices cucumber

Method:
Mix the honey and oatmeal together till thick. Adjust the proportions if necessary. Apply as a face pack and place the cucumber on your eyes. Rest for half an hour then wash off.

OATMEAL AND HONEY CLEANSER

This is a recipe made entirely from ingredients from the store cupboard. The choice of olive oil or vinegar for mixing is up to you and your skin type. Olive oil is best for normal to dry skin and vinegar if your skin tends to be on the greasy side. Don't use malt vinegar, however, which is chemically produced and won't smell nice, apart from possibly making your skin smart. Cider vinegar or any mild fruit vinegar would be best. You don't need much, anyway. It will keep for up to three months, so you could increase the proportions, but I think it is best to make just enough for one application.

You will need:
 1 tablespoon finely ground oats
 1 tablespoon wheat bran
 1 tablespoon honey
 Olive oil or cider vinegar to form a paste

Method:
Mix the oatmeal, wheat bran and honey together in a bowl. Add enough olive oil or cider vinegar to form a paste. Rinse your face with warm water, apply the cleanser and massage it gently into the skin. Rinse with warm water then splash your face with cold water.

SIMPLE OATMEAL AND HONEY CLEANSER

This simple mask takes advantage of the cleansing and softening properties of oats and the hydrating properties of honey.

You will need:
>   3 tablespoons oatmeal
>   2 tablespoons clear honey

Method:
Put the two ingredients in a bowl and stir well. The mixture will be quite stiff. Apply to a clean face and relax for about 15 minutes. Rinse well with warm water, depositing the oats in a bin.

OATMEAL CLEANSER FOR SENSITIVE SKIN

You will need:
>   240 ml (8 fluid oz) warm water
>   120 g (4 oz) oatmeal
>   1 tablespoon honey

Method:
Put all of the ingredients into a blender bowl and process until smooth. Place a little of the mixture on your palms and gently massage into your skin. Rinse with more warm water and pat dry.

STRAWBERRY AND HONEY FACE SCRUB

You will need:
>   4 medium-sized strawberries
>   60 g (2 oz) oatmeal, uncooked
>   3 teaspoons honey
>   2 teaspoons green tea

Method:
Wash and hull the strawberries. Blend the oatmeal, strawberries, green tea and honey. Apply a small amount to the skin, avoiding the eyes and using fingertips and

circular motions to work into the skin. Repeat until the face and neck are covered. Rinse completely, using lukewarm water. Store the remaining scrub in a covered container in the fridge for up to a week.

ROSE OIL AND HONEY MASK

You will need:

  2 tablespoons honey
  2 tablespoons sweet almond oil
  5 drops essential oil of rose
  1 drop vitamin E oil

Method:
Mix the honey and oils. Massage onto the face and neck with fingertips. Relax for 15 minutes, then rinse off with lukewarm water.

GREEN HONEY MASK

Maybe this is better for Halloween! Alternatively you could try this with a friend and see who makes the best scary face.

You will need:

  1 small packet fresh spinach, washed
  4 tablespoons fresh mint
  3 tablespoons honey
  1 teaspoon fresh ginger, crushed
  1 ripe banana
  2 egg whites

Method:
Blend the spinach, mint and ginger together. Add the honey and banana and blend until you have a liquid consistency. Add the egg whites and mix thoroughly. Apply a small amount to the entire face

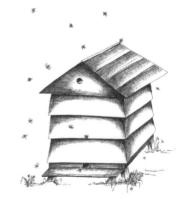

and neck, except the eyes. Allow to remain on the skin for 15 to 20 minutes while you take pictures to scare people with. Rinse and apply moisturiser.

APPLE TONER

You will need:

> 1 tablespoon honey
> 1 apple, peeled and cored

Method:
In a blender, purée the honey and apple. Smooth over the face and leave on for 15 minutes. Rinse with cool water.

HONEY LIP BALM

This might be a nice present for friends, as the amount you make would take ages to use, or you could halve the quantities. Be very careful with hot beeswax.

You will need:

> 225 ml (8 fluid oz) sweet almond oil
> 110 g (4 oz) beeswax
> 2 tablespoons honey

Method:
Place the almond oil and beeswax in a microwave-safe bowl. Microwave on high for about one minute, until the mixture melts. Whisk the honey into the wax. When cool, pour into small containers with lids. Apply to lips as a moisturiser or on top of lipstick for extra shine.

SKIN SOFTENING BATH

For a classically simple treat, try adding three or four tablespoons of honey to the bath water. You will enjoy a silky, fragrant bath.

FOAMING HONEY BATH

You will need: (enough for 4 baths)
    225 ml (8 fluid oz) sweet almond oil,
      light olive or sesame oil
    175 g (6 oz) honey
    100 g (3.5 oz) liquid soap
    1 tablespoon vanilla extract

Method:
Put the oil into a medium bowl and carefully stir in remaining ingredients until fully blended. Pour into a clean plastic bottle with a lid. Shake gently before using. Pour under running water and enjoy a warm, silky escape.

LAVENDER-HONEY MILK BATH

The lavender can be gathered from the garden after flowering on a dry day. The easiest way is to hang the flower heads upside down in a paper bag and hang in a dry place. As the seeds ripen they will be contained in the bag and you won't end up with lavender all over the place.

You will need: (makes 2 baths)
    3 tablespoons dried lavender flowers
    350 ml (12 fluid oz) whole milk or cream
    100 g (3.5 oz) honey

Method:
You can process the lavender flowers in a blender until they become a powder, or grind them in a mortar and pestle. Whisk together this lavender powder, milk and honey and then pour into a jar and seal. Before use, shake the jar and pour half of the mixture under running water. Store covered in the refrigerator for up to a week.

If you prefer something a little more adventurous or strenuous, you might like to consider one of these:

CHOCOLATE HONEY SCRUB

The original recipe calls for 225 g (8 oz) salt, which seems rather excessive. You could leave this ingredient out all together for a smooth consistency or gradually add the salt until you get to the texture you require.

You will need:
>   3 tablespoons cocoa powder
>   225 ml (8 fluid oz) honey
>   50 ml (2 fluid oz) oil

Method:
Mix the honey and oil together and stir in the cocoa. Gently massage all over before rinsing in the shower or bath.

MORNING BODY SCRUB

You will need:
>   50 g (2 oz) freshly ground coffee
>   50 ml (2 fluid oz) skimmed milk
>   2 tablespoons wheat germ
>   2 tablespoons honey
>   1 tablespoon grape seed or light oil
>   1 egg white

Method:
Mix together the milk, honey, oil and egg white. Slowly add the coffee and wheat germ, avoiding lumps. The

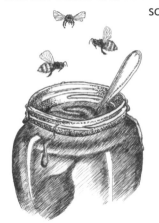

scrub should be even with a slightly gritty texture. Allow to stand. Apply all over in the shower or bath, using a body sponge to aid in exfoliation. Rinse off and dry. Apply your favourite moisturiser. Any remaining scrub can be kept for a day or two.

HAIR CONDITIONER

You will need:

120 ml (4 fluid oz) honey
2 tablespoons olive oil

Method:
Mix the honey and olive oil. Work a small amount at a time through the hair until coated. Cover the hair and leave on for 30 minutes. Shampoo well and rinse.

HAIR SHINE

You will need:

1 teaspoon honey
1 litre (1¾ pints) warm water

Method:
Stir the honey into warm water. After shampooing and rinsing, pour the mixture through your hair. Do not rinse out.

ROSEMARY HONEY HAIR CONDITIONER

You will need: For normal hair

120 ml (4 fluid oz) honey
2 tablespoons olive oil
4 drops essential oil of rosemary

Method:
Mix all the ingredients thoroughly. Pour into a clean plastic bottle with a lid. Apply a small amount at a time to slightly dampened hair before washing. Massage the scalp and work the mixture through the hair. Cover with a warm towel and leave for 30 minutes while you have a relaxing bath. Shampoo lightly and rinse with cool water.

HONEY AND MINT FEET TREAT

This is perfect for restoring the circulation after a long day on the go. It moisturises and softens tired, aching feet.

You will need:

- 4 tablespoons aloe vera gel
- 4 teaspoons grated beeswax
- 2 teaspoons honey
- 2 teaspoons freshly chopped mint, optional
- 6 drops peppermint essential oil
- 2 drops arnica oil
- 2 drops camphor oil
- 2 drops eucalyptus oil

Method:
Melt the beeswax in a microwave and combine with the aloe vera and honey. Add the mint and oils, stirring until completely mixed. Apply after a bath or shower to the feet and toes. Store the remaining mixture in a cool place.

SMOOTHING SKIN LOTION

You will need:

- 1 teaspoon honey
- 1 teaspoon vegetable oil
- ¼ teaspoon lemon juice

Method:
Mix all the ingredients together. Rub into hands, elbows, heels and any other areas of dry skin. Leave on for 10 minutes. Rinse off with warm water.

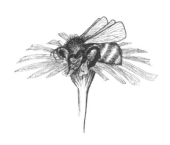

Culinary Uses
of Honey

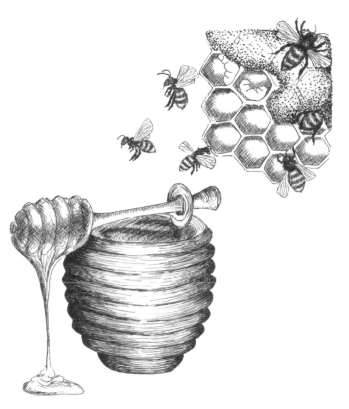

DRINKS

Honey can be used instead of sugar or sweetener to sweeten any drink. Bear in mind, though, that the type of honey you use may well add subtle flavours to your beverages. The following selection is just a starting point, especially when it comes to making refreshing fruit punches — something children love to do. A piece of fruit to garnish a simple, alcohol-free, fruit cocktail looks very grown up and exotic!

BREAKFAST DRINKS AND SMOOTHIES

HONEYED BEVERAGES

ALCOHOL-FREE JUICES AND PUNCHES

MULLED WINES, CIDERS, PUNCH

AND FESTIVE DRINKS

COCKTAILS

BREAKFAST DRINKS AND SMOOTHIES
Here's the perfect way to start the day with a fruit fix.
You can adjust the recipes to suit seasonal or personal
options.

HONEY STRAWBERRY SMOOTHIE

You will need: 4 servings

570 ml (1 pint) vanilla frozen yoghurt
1 punnet strawberries, hulled
240 ml (8 fluid oz) skimmed milk
2 tablespoons honey

Method:
Combine all the ingredients in a blender and process until
smooth.

GINGER PEACH SMOOTHIE

You will need: 4 servings

240 ml (8 fluid oz) boiling water
1 small cube fresh ginger root, peeled and crushed
2 tablespoons honey
2 fresh peaches, peeled and chopped
570 ml (1 pint) peach sorbet
1 tablespoon lime juice

Method:
1. Put the ginger in the hot water with the honey and
leave until cool.
2. Blend the peaches, sorbet and lime juice, then strain
the ginger and honey
water, adding to the
blender.
3. Process until you
have a smooth
smoothie.

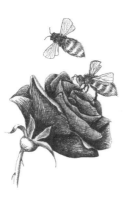

LOW-FAT BERRY MILKSHAKE

You will need: 4 servings

570 ml (1 pint) low-fat vanilla ice cream or
   low-fat frozen yoghurt
1 punnet strawberries, or assorted berries
   (e.g. raspberries, blueberries)
120 ml (4 fluid oz) skimmed milk
2 tablespoons honey
Mint sprigs (optional)

Method:
1. Put all of the ingredients except the mint into a
blender. Blend until creamy.
2. Serve immediately in tall, chilled glasses with a mint
sprig.

SUNRISE HEALTH DRINK

You will need: 4 servings

2 bananas
570 ml (1 pint) orange juice
2 small pots vanilla or plain yoghurt
2 tablespoons honey
2 dates, pitted

Method:
Blend all of the ingredients for approximately 1 minute.
Add more orange juice if necessary.

BANANA SMOOTHIE

You will need: 4 servings

570 ml (1 pint) skimmed milk
2 ripe bananas
2 small pots plain yoghurt
2 tablespoons honey
½ teaspoon ground cinnamon
Pinch of ground nutmeg
Ice cubes

Method:
1. Blend all of the ingredients except the ice for approximately 1 minute.
2. Add the ice cubes one at a time and blend until smooth.

PEAR AND YOGHURT SHAKE

You will need: Makes 4 servings

    1 large can (425 g, 15 oz) pears
    240 ml (8 fluid oz) plain low-fat yoghurt
    1 banana, peeled
    2 tablespoons honey
    Pinch of ground nutmeg

Method:
1. Mix the pears with juice, yoghurt, banana and honey in a blender until smooth.
2. Pour into chilled glasses, sprinkle with nutmeg and serve immediately.

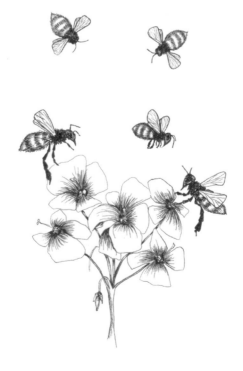

HONEYED BEVERAGES

CHAI (SPICED INDIAN TEA)

You will need for the base: Makes 4 cups

570 ml (1 pint) water
2 black tea bags
2 teaspoons vanilla extract
½ teaspoon ground ginger
½ teaspoon ground cinnamon
½ teaspoon ground allspice
120 ml (4 fluid oz) honey
Milk to taste

Method:
1. Combine the spices, honey and water in a saucepan and bring to the boil. Add the tea bags and leave to steep for 5 minutes.
2. Remove the tea bags. Cover and refrigerate.

To serve hot: combine the base with milk to taste in a saucepan or microwave.
To serve cold: combine the base, with or without milk, over ice cubes.

MEXICAN COFFEE

You will need: Makes 4 cups

4 cups hot espresso-style coffee
200 ml (7 fluid oz) milk
120 ml (4 fluid oz) honey
2 tablespoons cocoa powder
1 teaspoon ground cinnamon
Sweetened whipped cream
Chocolate shavings

Method:
1. Combine the cocoa powder and cinnamon with a little milk and the honey to form a paste.
2. Add the coffee and milk. Pour into mugs; garnish with whipped cream and chocolate shavings.

SPICED CAMOMILE COOLER

You can add a tablespoon of orange juice to each glass as a variation.

You will need: Makes 4 servings

570 ml (1 pint) water
4 camomile tea bags
4 cinnamon sticks
16 whole cloves
120 ml (4 fluid oz) honey
110 ml (2 fluid oz) fresh lemon juice
Orange juice (optional)

Method:
1. Bring the water to the boil in a medium saucepan. Add the tea bags, cinnamon and cloves, and simmer for 5 minutes.
2. Remove the tea bags, cinnamon and cloves and stir in the honey and lemon juice.
3. Chill thoroughly. Pour over ice and garnish with fresh lemon slices.

SPICED HONEY ECHINACEA SOOTHER

You will need: Makes 4 servings

4 echinacea tea bags
4 cinnamon sticks
8 cloves
120 ml (4 fluid oz) honey
120 ml (4 fluid oz) fresh lemon juice

Method:
1. Place a tea bag, a cinnamon stick and two cloves in each mug. Fill three-quarters full with boiling water and steep for 5 minutes.
2. Remove the tea bag, cinnamon and cloves, and stir in the honey and lemon juice.

ICED HONEY TEA

You will need: Makes 4 servings

570 ml (1 pint) boiling water
4 tea bags
Juice of ½ lemon
120 ml (4 fluid oz) honey
Mint sprigs, optional

Method:
1. Add the boiled water to the tea bags and allow to infuse for 5 minutes.
2. Remove tea bags and add the lemon juice and honey. Stir well.
3. Chill thoroughly and serve over ice cubes in tall glasses. Garnish with mint if desired.

SPICED HONEY COFFEE

You will need: Makes 4 cups

2 tablespoons honey
4 whole cloves
4 cinnamon sticks
Peel of ½ lemon
60 ml (2 fluid oz) brandy
Strong hot coffee

Method:
1. Put the honey, cloves, cinnamon sticks and lemon peel into a small saucepan. Cook and stir over a medium heat until this mixture boils.
2. Stir in the brandy. Put 1 tablespoon of the mixture into each cup or mug and top up with hot coffee.

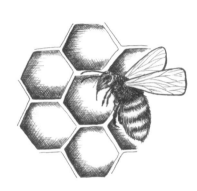

ALCOHOL-FREE JUICES AND PUNCHES

A really impressive thing to do for parties is to freeze small leaves of herbs, such as mint, or small fruit, such as cranberries, in ice cubes. Obviously you have to think ahead, but once made they can be added to cold drinks at the last minute, or offered to surprise guests in a quick drink.

Hot punches may cause problems if you try to pour very hot liquid into glasses. There's also the danger of scalding or burning your guests, who may not be aware that the drink you are offering is hot. That has happened to me more than once at parties, so watch out!

HOT FRUIT AND HONEY PUNCH

You will need: Makes 8 servings

570 ml (1 pint) apple juice
570 ml (1 pint) cranberry juice
60 ml (2 fluid oz) honey
1 cinnamon stick
½ lemon, sliced
6 whole cloves

Method:
1. Heat the apple juice with the honey, spices and lemon, but don't allow it to boil.
2. Add the cranberry juice, stirring to combine, and heat gently.
3. Pour carefully into serving glasses or mugs.

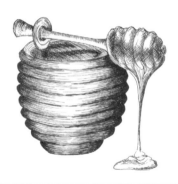

TROPICAL JUICE QUENCHER

You could make ice cubes with extra lime juice to add a bit of extra sparkle.
Slices of fresh orange and/or limes also look good.

You will need: Makes 4 to 6 servings
   200 ml (7 fluid oz) pineapple juice
   200 ml (7 fluid oz) orange juice
   60 ml (2 fluid oz) lime juice
   60 ml (2 fluid oz) clear honey
   570 ml (1 pint) sparkling mineral water

Method:
1. Mix the honey and a small amount of juice together in a jug until the honey is dissolved.
2. Chill until ready to serve. Just before serving, stir in sparkling water and ice (optional).

PINK DRINK

You will need: Makes 4 servings
   1 small punnet strawberries
   2 ripe bananas
   240 ml (8 fluid oz) orange juice
   2 tablespoons honey
   Ice cubes

Method:
1. Put the fruit, juice, honey and ice into a blender for 15 seconds on high speed.
2. Stir the ingredients with a spatula and blend for a further 15 seconds.
3. Serve chilled in a glass with slices of strawberry and banana speared on a cocktail stick.

PARTY PUNCH

The first part of this can be prepared well in advance, with just the finishing ingredients to add when your guests have arrived.

A large punch bowl looks really good, but if you haven't got one you can improvise with a couple of large jugs or even a clean washing-up bowl or mixing bowl.

You will need: Serves 10 to 12

570 ml (1 pint) boiling water
120 ml (4 fluid oz) honey
1 litre (1¾ pints) cranberry juice
570 ml (1 pint) orange juice
240 ml (8 fluid oz) lemon juice
1 litre (1¾ pints) ginger ale
Ice cubes

Method:
1. Dissolve the honey in the boiling water and leave to chill.
2. In a large bowl combine the juices. Stir in the honey mixture.
3. Just before serving add the ginger ale and ice cubes. Garnish with fruit.

ORANGE JUICER

You will need: Makes 2 servings

60 ml (2 fluid oz) honey
1 small can concentrated orange juice
240 ml (8 fluid oz) milk
6 ice cubes

Method:
1. Put the honey, juice and ice cubes in a blender. Process until smooth.
2. Add the milk and serve.

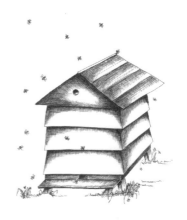

PINEAPPLE PUNCH

You will need: Makes 4 servings

570 ml (1 pint) pineapple juice
60 ml (2 fluid oz) fresh lime juice
60 ml (2 fluid oz) honey
1 lime, thinly sliced
570 ml (1 pint) sparkling mineral water

Method:
1. Mix the juices, honey and lime slices in a jug and put in the fridge until required.
2. Add the mineral water and serve straight away.

CRANBERRY PUNCH

I served this last Christmas at a party. It was an instant hit with the drivers among the guests, and I don't think they missed the alcohol! It looks more adult than the orange-based varieties.

You will need:

60 ml (2 fluid oz) honey
120 ml (4 fluid oz) orange juice
1 litre (1¾ pints) sparkling mineral water
200 ml (7 fluid oz) cranberry juice
4 tablespoons tap water
1 stick cinnamon
1 small orange
Fresh cranberries and mint to garnish
    or make into ice cubes (optional)

Method:
1. Put the orange juice, honey and cinnamon with the tap water in a small pan. Heat gently to melt the honey, then boil briefly. Leave to cool.
2. When ready to serve, put the cranberry juice, mineral water and slices of orange into a punch bowl with the prepared syrup. Add the cranberries and leaves of mint or prepared ice cubes.

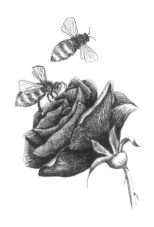

MULLED APPLE JUICE

You will need: Makes 4 to 6 servings

Juice of 1 lemon
1 orange, cut in half
12 whole cloves
1 litre (1¾ pints) apple juice
120 ml (4 fluid oz) honey
2 cinnamon sticks
¼ teaspoon ground ginger

Method:
1. Stick the cloves into the orange pieces.
2. Stir the lemon juice, apple juice and honey over a low heat. Add the cinnamon sticks, ginger and orange pieces.
3. Bring to the boil over a medium heat and serve carefully in heatproof containers.

MULLED WINES, CIDERS, PUNCH AND FESTIVE DRINKS

Christmas and New Year are the special times for mulled wines, although the chilled versions are quite refreshing in hot weather. A French friend surprised us last summer with a white wine equivalent which packed quite a punch!

Honey seems to be a natural complement to red wine, cloves and cinnamon in a number of countries, probably because these ingredients evoke the smell of mead and medieval winter festivals.

MULLED RED WINE

The good thing about this is you can keep adding to it as the need arises. You don't have to use good wine either, as the other ingredients soften even the roughest red. The addition of water means that everyone can enjoy it for longer, without getting pickled. I added Cointreau last year, because we had some left over.

You will need: Makes 12 servings

- 2 bottles cheap red wine
- 1.5 litres (2½ pints) water
- 6 tablespoons honey
- 1 stick cinnamon
- 3 oranges
- 2 lemons
- 2 teaspoons grated fresh root ginger
- 12 cloves
- 2 tablespoons brandy or liqueur (optional)

Method:

1. Stick the cloves into one of the oranges, all over the outside.
2. Put all the ingredients into a large saucepan and heat to simmering point. Don't let it boil.
3. Simmer for 20 minutes, stirring occasionally. Serve immediately (with a warning about the heat!).

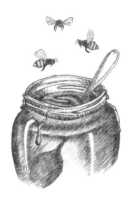

HOT HONEY CIDER

Again, once the spices are doing their job, you can add extra cider to this recipe, as required.

You will need: Makes 8 to 10 servings

  2 litres (3½ pints) apple cider
  240 ml (8 fluid oz) honey
  120 ml (4 fluid oz) orange juice
  Juice of ½ lemon
  3 cinnamon sticks
  2 teaspoons whole cloves
  ¼ teaspoon allspice
  1 apple
  1 orange
  240 ml (8 fluid oz) rum, optional

Method:
1. Put the cider, honey, orange juice, lemon juice, cinnamon sticks, cloves and allspice into a large saucepan. Simmer on medium-low heat for 20 minutes.
2. Slice the apple and orange thinly, leaving the core and peels. Add to pot with rum, if required. Serve warm.

VINEYARD PUNCH

You will need: Makes 8 to 10 servings

  1 bottle cheap red wine
  570 ml (1 pint) apple juice
  120 ml (4 fluid oz) honey
  1 small punnet strawberries
  1 small lime, sliced
  240 ml (8 fluid oz) ginger ale
  Ice cubes

Method:
1. Mix the wine, apple juice and honey in a large jug or bowl. Add lime slices and strawberries.
2. Chill until required. Just before serving, add the ginger ale and serve over ice cubes in tall glasses. Garnish each glass with some of the fruit.

SPICED ALE

You will need: Makes 4 to 6 servings

1 litre (1¾ pints) ale
2 glasses brandy
Peel of 1 lemon
Pinch of nutmeg
120 ml (4 fluid oz) honey

Method:
1. Place all the ingredients except the brandy in a saucepan and simmer, but don't allow to boil.
2. Add the brandy and serve immediately.

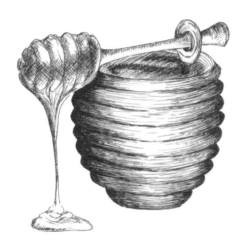

COCKTAILS

Honey has a place in many well-known cocktails. Here are a few starters. Making up a quantity of honey syrup before you start will make things easier. Use a shot glass or measuring jug, rather than just hoping for the best, and remember that there is a significant alcohol content in each drink! Quantities are based on each cocktail, so 25 ml is equivalent to 1 fluid ounce.

If you have a cocktail shaker that was given to you as a Christmas or birthday present, this could be the time to use it. If not, a jug or screw-top jar will do for mixing.

HONEY SYRUP BASE

You will need:

> Honey
> Boiling water

Method:
Mix 4 parts honey to 1 part hot water and cool before use.

PINK HONEY BEE

You will need:

> 2 parts vodka or rum
> 1 part honey syrup
> 3 parts cranberry juice

Method:
Shake with ice and strain into a large cocktail glass. Garnish with a cherry.

PASSION POTION

You will need:

> 2 parts pink grapefruit juice
> 1 part honey syrup
> 1 part rum or vodka
> Ice cubes

Method:
Combine grapefruit juice and honey syrup. Fill a glass with ice. Pour the rum over the ice and add the grapefruit juice mixture.

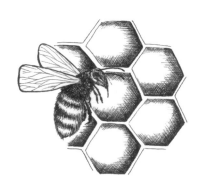

KENTUCKY COOLER

You will need:

 1 part whisky
 ½ shot Triple Sec (or Cointreau)
 2 parts honey syrup
 1 part iced tea
 1 part ginger ale
 2 lemon wedges

Method:
Build this in the glass over ice cubes.

GOLDEN HONEY MARGARITA

You will need:

 1 part tequila
 ½ shot Triple Sec (or Cointreau)
 1 part honey syrup
 2 parts lemon juice
 Salt

Method:
Shake well with ice, and strain into a large cocktail glass
with a salted rim.

HONEY MINT JULEPS

The easiest way to make the mint syrup is to make it as
for honey syrup, adding the leaves of mint and allowing it
to cool, then straining it to remove the leaves. Save a
few sprigs of fresh mint for a garnish.

You will need:

 Sprigs of mint
 1 part honey mint syrup
 1 part bourbon
 Ice

Method:
Combine the bourbon with the honey mint syrup. Pour over crushed ice into a frosted tumbler or tall glass. Garnish with mint sprigs.

MANDARIN BLOSSOM

You could substitute the flavour of the vodka or use plain vodka.

You will need:

    1 part honey syrup
    2 parts lemon juice
    1 part mandarin-flavoured vodka
    1 tablespoon egg white, for froth (optional)
    Cinnamon and icing sugar for rimming the glass

Method:
Shake all ingredients with ice. Strain into a cinnamon-sugar-rimmed glass.

MOJITO HONITO

You will need:
    1 part honey mint syrup (see page 101)
    1 part freshly squeezed lime juice
    2 to 3 fresh mint leaves
    1 part light rum
    3 parts soda water

Method:
Combine the honey mint syrup and a splash of soda water in a tall glass. Add the lime and rum. Stir and fill with ice. Top with soda water and garnish with a mint sprig or lime wedge.

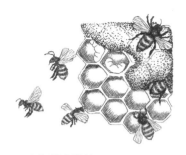

HAPPY HONEY COCKTAIL

You will need:

> 1 part brandy
> 1 part grapefruit juice
> 1 part honey syrup
> Ice

Method:
Shake the liquids together and pour over ice cubes

HONEY RUM STINGER

You will need:

> 1 part dark rum
> 3 drops Angostura Bitters
> 1 teaspoon honey
> 1 part lime juice
> Ice

Method:
Mix together and pour over the crushed ice.

BUMBLE BEE

You will need:

> 2 parts dark rum
> 1 part honey syrup
> 1 part lemon juice
> Ice

Method:
Mix together and pour over the crushed ice.

WHISKY HONEY CREAM

You will need:

    2 parts whisky
    1 part double cream
    1 part honey syrup
    Ice

Method:

Mix together and pour over the crushed ice.

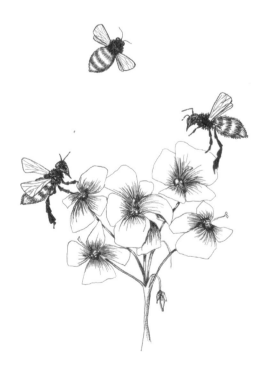

SAUCES AND MARINADES

SAUCES AND MARINADES

The easiest way to make most of these dressings is to use a clean, screw-topped jar in which to mix the ingredients in. The leftovers can be kept in the fridge in most cases, for some weeks, unless dairy products are involved. It's a handy way of always having some salad dressing at the ready to encourage you to eat more salad. The honey you use can make all the difference to the flavour, so beware when using strongly flavoured varieties. On removing dressing from the fridge it will look cloudy, but don't worry: let it reach room temperature and shake again.

EVERYDAY FRENCH DRESSING

You will need:

175 ml (6 fluid oz) olive oil
4 tablespoons wine vinegar
1 teaspoon French mustard
1 clove of garlic
1 teaspoon clear honey
Salt and pepper

Shake together in a jar and serve.

SWEET AND SOUR SALAD DRESSING

You will need:
60 ml (2 fluid oz) honey
40 ml (2½ tablespoons) rice wine vinegar
1 tablespoon diced onion
¼ teaspoon garlic salt
Salt and pepper
120 ml (8 tablespoons) olive oil

Combine the honey, vinegar, onion, salts and pepper and blend until smooth. Pour in the oil in a slow, steady stream and mix until smooth, or use a screw-top jar to shake and mix.

MINT AND HONEY DRESSING

You will need:

3 tablespoons olive oil
4 tablespoons cider vinegar
2 tablespoons clear honey
1 tablespoon chopped, fresh mint
Salt and pepper

Shake together until blended. This goes well with watercress salad.

HONEY HERB DRESSING (FAT-FREE)

You will need:

60 ml (2 fluid oz) honey
60 ml (2 fluid oz) white wine vinegar
2 tablespoons chopped fresh basil
1 tablespoon spring onion
Salt and pepper, to taste

Combine all ingredients and mix well.

ALL-PURPOSE HONEY DRESSING

You will need:

120 ml (4 fluid oz) balsamic vinegar
60 ml (2 fluid oz) honey
2 tablespoons olive oil
1 tablespoon favourite fresh herb

Mix all ingredients together and use to coat a green salad or fresh fruit salad.

CINNAMON GINGER DRESSING

You will need:

2.5 cm (1 in) fresh root ginger, grated
3 tablespoons olive oil
1 tablespoon white wine vinegar
1 tablespoon honey
½ teaspoon ground cinnamon
Salt and black pepper

Combine all ingredients and mix well.

HONEY, ORANGE AND YOGHURT DRESSING

You will need:

3 tablespoons honey
1 small pot plain yoghurt
50 g (2 oz) mayonnaise
3 tablespoons orange juice
1 teaspoon cider vinegar
1 teaspoon grated orange peel
¼ teaspoon dry mustard

Method:
1. Mix the honey, yoghurt, mayonnaise, dry mustard and orange peel.
2. Gradually mix in the orange juice and vinegar.

HONEY BARBECUE SAUCE

This can be used to marinate beef, chicken or pork before cooking. Alternatively, serve as a sauce with barbecued meat or vegetables.

You will need:

50 g (2 oz) minced onion
1 clove of garlic, crushed or finely sliced
1 tablespoon vegetable oil
50 g (2 oz) tomato purée
120 ml (4 fluid oz) honey
2 tablespoons vinegar

2 tablespoons minced parsley
1 tablespoon Worcestershire sauce
Black pepper
Pinch cayenne pepper

Method:
1. Sauté the onion and garlic in oil until browned.
2. Add the remaining ingredients and bring the mixture to the boil.
3. Reduce heat and simmer for 5 minutes. Cool before using as a marinade.

ORANGE-HONEY MARINADE

Very spicy!

You will need:
6 tablespoons honey
6 tablespoons soy sauce
275 ml (10 fluid oz) orange juice
3 tablespoons water
150 ml (5 fluid oz) dry white wine
1 teaspoon mustard
1 teaspoon paprika
½ teaspoon allspice
1 clove of garlic, crushed
¼ teaspoon tabasco sauce

Combine all the ingredients and leave to stand for at least 20 minutes to allow the flavours to develop. Use to marinate pork or chicken. It will also spice up vegetables in a stir-fry.

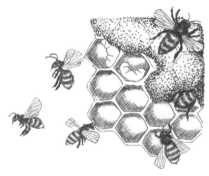

ORIENTAL DIPPING SAUCE

You will need:

120 ml (4 fluid oz) honey
50 g (2 oz) peanut butter
1 tablespoon soy sauce
1 clove of garlic, crushed
1 teaspoon freshly chopped coriander

Place all the ingredients in a bowl and mix well. Use to dip cooked items in, e.g. chicken shreds, before eating.

HONEY AND THYME MUSTARD

You will need:

225 g (8 oz) Dijon mustard
120 ml (4 fluid oz) honey
1 teaspoon crushed dried thyme or fresh leaves

Whisk together all ingredients in small bowl until well blended. Refrigerate until ready to use.

HOMEMADE HONEY MUSTARD

You will need:

225 g (8 oz) white mustard seeds
275 ml (10 fluid oz) white wine vinegar
1 teaspoon ground cinnamon
60 ml (2 fluid oz) honey

Method:
1. Place the mustard seeds, vinegar and cinnamon in a bowl, cover and leave to soak overnight.
2. Pound together with the honey with a mortar and pestle until you get a thick paste, or blend in a processor. Add more vinegar if it is too stiff.
3. Transfer to sterilised jars, cover and store in the fridge for up to one month.

SWEET AND SOUR SAUCE

You will need:

120 ml (4 fluid oz) honey
1 tablespoon cornflour
80 ml (3 fluid oz) red wine vinegar
80 ml (3 fluid oz) chicken stock
1 green pepper, finely chopped
2 tablespoons pimentos, chopped
1 tablespoon soy sauce
¼ teaspoon garlic powder
¼ teaspoon ground ginger

In a saucepan, combine honey and cornflour. Stir in the
vinegar, chicken stock and the other ingredients. Simmer
for about 20 to 30 minutes.

ORIENTAL MARINADE AND BASTE FOR BEEF

You will need:

4 tablespoons white wine
150 ml (¼ pint) chicken broth
75 ml (5 tablespoons) soy sauce
⅛ teaspoon garlic powder
3 tablespoons wine vinegar
2 tablespoons honey

Shake all ingredients together in a screw-top jar.
Marinate strips of steak for several hours in the sauce
before grilling. Baste meat with the sauce while cooking.

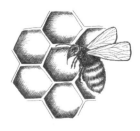

DESSERT SAUCES

HONEY LIME CREAM DRESSING

You will need: Makes 1 cup

½ cup whipping cream
2 tablespoons honey
1 teaspoon grated lime peel

Beat whipping cream until fluffy. Drizzle in honey and beat until stiff. Fold in grated lime peel. Serve over ice cream.

ALMOND AND HONEY BRICKLE

You will need:

2 tablespoons melted butter
60 ml (2 fluid oz) honey
200 g (7 oz) slivered almonds
Pinch of salt
6 tablespoons cream

Method:
1. Put the butter and honey in a saucepan over a medium-high heat. Add the almonds and stir constantly for about 5 to 6 minutes until it darkens to a rich caramel. Do not leave unattended, as the mixture will burn easily.
2. Remove from the heat and add the salt and stir the cream in slowly. The mixture will sputter and steam, so use a long-handled spoon and keep face and hands away.
3. Pour the sauce into a bowl and allow to cool. Serve with ice cream or a steamed pudding.

For an easy clean-up, add about 2.5 cm (1 in) of water to the pan and bring to a simmer for about 5 minutes to loosen the caramel.

STARTERS AND APPETISERS

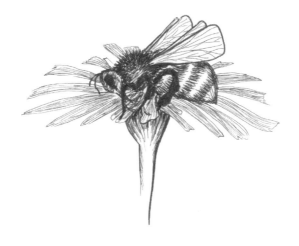

GOAT'S CHEESE '*AMUSE-GUEULE*'

These are a regular favourite with *aperitifs* in France, where the drinks and conversation are the main event, but you really need more than a few crisps or olives to sustain you until the first course arrives. Such a social gathering has been known to last way beyond the customary two drinks, in my experience, and I always need something to sustain me! They seem to go down well here in the UK, too. The French sell goat's cheese in a longish roll, which is ideal for slicing into 12 to 15 thin slices. If you can't find the roll variety, use wedges from a circular cheese. Allow 3 to 4 slices of bread per person. It doesn't matter if the bread is stale: in fact it's a good way of avoiding waste.

You will need:

> 1 thin French baguette (or flûte)
> Goat's cheese
> Clear honey
> Olive oil

Method:

1. Slice the goat's cheese thinly and preheat the grill.
2. Slice the bread thinly and brush with olive oil on both sides. Place all of the required bread under a hot grill until the bread just starts to brown, but don't let it burn. Lightly toast the second side.
3. Put a piece of cheese onto each round of baguette and return to the grill until the cheese starts to melt and bubble.

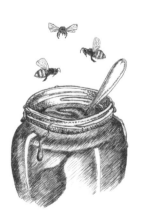

4. Remove to a plate and drizzle the honey over the cheese. Serve immediately. You won't have any leftovers!

HONEY-GRILLED SCALLOPS

You will need: Serves 4

12 scallops, prepared and washed (if frozen, thaw
   thoroughly)
2 tablespoons lime juice
1 tablespoon vegetable oil
1 tablespoon honey
1 tablespoon soy sauce
1 teaspoon finely grated root ginger

Method:
1. Place the lime juice, oil, honey, soy sauce and ginger
in a bowl and mix well.
2. Add the scallops, toss to coat thoroughly then cover
and refrigerate for 1 hour.
3. Preheat the grill to hot. Remove the scallops from the
bowl, reserving the marinade and place in a grill pan
which has been lightly oiled. Grill for 3 to 4 minutes then
turn and baste with reserved marinade and continue
grilling for a further 3 to 4 minutes or until opaque
throughout. Serve immediately on a bed of salad leaves.

PEPPERED FETA

You will need: Serves 4

Mixed salad leaves
450 g (1 lb) feta cheese
3 teaspoons coarsely ground black pepper
80 ml (3 fluid oz) honey
Slices of French bread to serve

Method:
1. Pat the feta cheese dry, cut into cubes and arrange on
salad leaves in the centre of each plate.
2. Mix together the pepper and honey then drizzle the
mixture over the top of the feta cheese. Serve with the
bread slices.

ASPARAGUS WITH HONEY GARLIC SAUCE

You will need: Serves 4

   450 g (1 lb) fresh asparagus
   110 g (4 oz) Dijon mustard
   120 ml (4 fluid oz) dark ale beer
   4 tablespoons honey
   1 clove of garlic, finely chopped
   ½ teaspoon crushed thyme leaves
   ½ teaspoon salt

Method:
1. Steam or cook the asparagus in boiling water for about 2 minutes or until barely tender. Drain and cool.
2. Mix the mustard, ale, honey, garlic, thyme and salt. Pour over the cooled asparagus and serve.

ALMOND LETTUCE WEDGES WITH DRESSING

You will need:

   1 quantity of preferred or honey mustard dressing
     (see page 106)
   1 head iceberg lettuce
   110 g (4 oz) slivered or sliced almonds, toasted

Method:
1. Remove the core from lettuce, rinse and drain thoroughly. Cut into 6 wedges. Chill thoroughly.
2. Place on serving plates. Spoon over your favourite dressing. Just before serving, sprinkle the lettuce wedges with almonds.

HONEYED GORGONZOLA CROSTINI

A similar idea to the goat's cheese nibbles. If you don't like the rather strong taste of the cheese, this may be more to your liking. You get more honey and less olive oil.

You will need: Serves 4

    8 x 1 cm (½ in) slices baguette
    110 g (4 oz) mild Gorgonzola cheese
    8 teaspoons honey
    Baby salad leaves to serve

Method:

1. Preheat the grill and lightly toast both sides of the bread.
2. Divide the honey between the toasted bread, spread evenly on all pieces of bread.
3. Divide the Gorgonzola cheese between the slices evenly, then toast for a few minutes under the grill until the cheese has melted.
4. Place the salad leaves on 4 individual plates and then place 2 crostini on each plate and serve immediately.

HONEY-DRESSED COUSCOUS SALAD

You will need: Serves 4 to 6

    275 ml (10 fluid oz) water
    225 g (8 oz) couscous
    225 g (8 oz) shredded cooked chicken breast
    1 tin chickpeas, rinsed and drained
    2 medium carrots, grated
    3 spring onions, thinly sliced
    3 tablespoons finely chopped parsley

You will need for the dressing:

    4 tablespoons fresh lemon juice
    3 tablespoons honey
    2 tablespoons olive oil
    2 teaspoons freshly grated lemon peel
    Salt and freshly ground black pepper

Method:

1. In a small bowl or screw-top jar, combine dressing ingredients; mix until blended.
2. Bring the water to the boil. Remove from heat and stir in the couscous. Cover and let it stand for 5 minutes, then fluff with a fork. Remove to a large bowl and let it cool.
3. When ready to serve stir in the chicken, chickpeas, carrots, onion and parsley. Add the dressing, tossing to coat the salad.

SENEGALESE SOUP

This recipe calls for a combination of chicken, milk and shrimps, but I prefer to leave out the shrimps.

You will need: Serves 4

    1 tablespoon oil
    1 finely chopped onion
    1 tablespoon cornflour
    2 teaspoons curry powder
    2 tins chicken broth
    2 tablespoons fresh lime juice
    4 tablespoons honey
    225 g (8 oz) sweetcorn, fresh or frozen
    240 ml (8 fluid oz) milk
    225 g (8 oz) cooked shrimps (optional)
    Salt, optional

Method:
1. In a medium saucepan cook the onion in oil for 3 to 5 minutes or until tender. Stir in the curry powder; cook and stir for a minute.
2. Mix the cornflour with the lime juice and honey and add to the pan, stirring all the time. Whisk in the chicken broth and bring to the boil. Stir in the sweetcorn.
3. Reduce the heat and simmer for 3 minutes. Stir in milk and optional shrimps. Season if you wish.
4. Cool the soup, transfer to a bowl, cover and refrigerate for at least 2 hours, until well chilled.

CITRUS AND AVOCADO SALAD

This makes a refreshing change from my all-time standby of avocado and tomato salad. I recently tried a similar recipe with two small cooked beetroot and the juice of a lime instead of the grapefruit. This would use three superfoods, i.e. avocado, beetroot and orange, in the same recipe — bonus points there for healthy eating!

You will need: Serves 6

    3 x 15 cm (6 in) tortillas
    3 medium oranges
    2—3 grapefruits
    3 ripe avocados
    2 tablespoons honey
    2 tablespoons raspberry vinegar
    Sprigs of fresh mint

Method:

1. Slice the corn tortillas into very thin strips. Dry them by placing on a baking sheet and putting in a very cool oven 110°C (225°F, gas mark ¼) for approximately 15 minutes. Leave to cool.

2. Grate the orange rind to obtain approximately 2 teaspoons of orange rind for each serving. Peel the oranges and grapefruits, pull into segments and remove the pips. Prepare the avocados by removing skin and stones and cutting into slices lengthways.

3. In a large bowl mix the honey, raspberry vinegar, orange and grapefruit sections. Add the orange rinds and tortilla strips. Toss all of the ingredients gently. Top with avocado slices and a sprig of fresh mint for garnish.

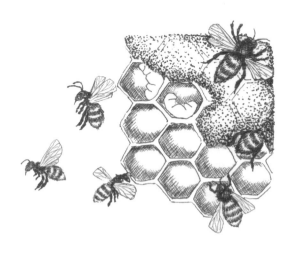

BUDAPEST BORTSCH

You will need: Serves 4

350 g (12 oz) red cabbage
2–3 beetroot
2–3 boiling potatoes
1 small tin tomatoes
1 tablespoon vegetable oil
1 onion, diced
1 clove of garlic, finely chopped
700 ml (24 fluid oz) water
4 tablespoons red wine vinegar
1 tablespoon honey
3 tablespoons parsley
1 teaspoon thyme
1 bay leaf
1 teaspoon dried dill
½ tablespoon Hungarian paprika
1 teaspoon salt
Freshly ground black pepper
4 tablespoons sour cream, for garnish
2 tablespoons fresh dill, for garnish (optional)

Method:
1. Slice the cabbage into thin strips. Peel the beetroot with a sharp knife and cut into strips. Peel the potatoes and cut in half.
2. In a large saucepan, heat the oil and sauté the onion and garlic for 5 minutes. Add the cabbage, beets, potatoes, tomatoes and all other ingredients except the sour cream and garnish. Bring to the boil and reduce heat. Simmer for at least 25 minutes.
3. Serve with a dollop of sour cream and a garnish of dill.

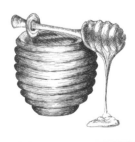

MAIN DISHES

Although honey is usually associated with desserts or drinks, there are some styles of cooking that call for a contrast of flavours, such as sweet and sour dishes. Here is a selection for you to drool over.

POULTRY DISHES

GINGER TURKEY STIR-FRY

You will need: Serves 4 to 6

  80 ml (3 fluid oz) water
  2 tablespoons fresh lemon juice
  2 tablespoons honey
  1 teaspoon freshly grated root ginger
  1 tablespoon light soy sauce
  1 large clove of garlic, minced
  2 tablespoons cornflour
  1 tablespoon vegetable oil
  2 medium carrots, diagonally sliced
  1 small head broccoli, cut into florets
  110 g (4 oz) mushrooms, sliced
  1 small can sliced water chestnuts
  450 g (1 lb) uncooked turkey breast, cut into strips

Method:
1. Mix the water, lemon juice, honey, ginger, soy sauce and garlic. Dissolve the cornflour in this mixture.
2. Heat the oil over a high heat in a wok or large skillet. Add the carrots and stir-fry for about 3 minutes or until tender. Add the broccoli, mushrooms and water chestnuts and stir-fry for about two more minutes. Remove from pan.
3. Stir-fry the turkey until lightly browned. Add the sauce and cook, stirring constantly, until thickened. Add the vegetables and heat them through. Serve immediately.

DUCK BREAST WITH TANGY HONEY SAUCE

You will need: Serves 4

  110 g (4 oz) canned crushed pineapple, undrained
  3 tablespoons honey
  4 tablespoons dry sherry or chicken broth
  4 tablespoons soy sauce
  4 tablespoons Worcestershire sauce
  1 tablespoon orange juice
  1 tablespoon cider vinegar
  1 clove of garlic, crushed
  4 duck breasts

Method:

1. Mix the pineapple, honey, sherry or chicken broth, soy sauce, Worcestershire sauce, orange juice, vinegar and garlic in a saucepan. Simmer over a low heat for an hour to blend the flavours.

2. Prick the duck breasts all over with a fork and sprinkle with pepper to taste. Arrange on a rack in a roasting pan and brush with butter. Roast at 200°C (400°F, gas mark 6) for about 40 minutes or until golden brown.

3. Serve with the sauce.

SWEET AND SOUR CHICKEN

You will need: Serves 4

    4 tablespoons rice vinegar

    2 tablespoons light soy sauce

    2 tablespoons vegetable oil

    2 tablespoons honey

    1 teaspoon freshly grated root ginger

    Pepper

    3—4 boneless, skinless chicken breasts

    3 onions, thinly sliced

    1 red pepper, cut into strips

    1 clove of garlic, crushed

    110 g (4 oz) chopped walnuts (optional)

Method:

1. Blend the vinegar with the soy sauce, oil, honey, ginger and pepper.

2. Slice the chicken into strips and marinate with the onions in some of the sauce for 15 minutes.

3. In a large skillet or wok, stir-fry the chicken with the onions, red pepper and garlic. Add the remaining sauce and heat through. Sprinkle on the walnuts.

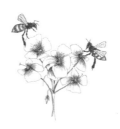

LEMON BASIL CHICKEN

You will need: Serves 4

    120 ml (4 fluid oz) honey
    4 tablespoons lemon juice
    1 tablespoon freshly chopped basil
    1 clove of garlic, crushed
    ½ teaspoon salt
    2 tablespoons grated lemon zest
    4 boneless, skinless chicken breasts

Method:

1. Put all of the ingredients apart from the chicken in a bowl and mix well.
2. Add the chicken breasts then cover and refrigerate for at least an hour. Turn during the marinating period.
3. Preheat the oven to 180°C (350°F, gas Mark 4). Transfer the marinated chicken to a shallow ovenproof dish and bake for 35 to 40 minutes or until thoroughly cooked. Garnish with a sprig of basil.

MOROCCAN CHICKEN TAJINE

You will need: Serves 4

    8 skinless chicken thighs
    3—4 tablespoons honey
    1 large onion, chopped
    3 cloves of garlic, crushed
    2 cinnamon sticks
    1 lemon
    2 teaspoons turmeric
    110 g (4 oz) dried apricots, quartered

Method:

1. Arrange the chicken thighs in a casserole dish. Pour over the honey and sprinkle with onion and garlic.
2. Add the cinnamon sticks and sprinkle with lemon juice and turmeric. Top with apricot quarters and bake in a moderate oven at 180°C (350°F, gas mark 4) for about 1 hour or until the chicken is tender.
3. Remove the cinnamon sticks from the casserole and serve with couscous.

MEAT DISHES

PORK STIR-FRY

You will need: Serves 4 to 6

450 g (1 lb) pork steak or loin
200 ml (7 fluid oz) orange juice
2 tablespoons honey
3 tablespoons soy sauce
1 tablespoon cornflour
¼ teaspoon ground ginger
2 tablespoons vegetable oil
2 carrots, diagonally cut
2 sticks celery, diagonally cut
110 g (4 oz) cashews or peanuts

Method:
1. Cut the pork into thin strips and set aside.
2. Mix the orange juice, honey, soy sauce, cornflour and ginger.
3. Heat 1 tablespoon oil in a wok or skillet over medium heat. Add the carrots and celery and stir-fry for about 3 minutes. Remove the vegetables.
4. Pour the remaining oil into the skillet, add the pork and stir-fry about 5 minutes or until thoroughly cooked.
5. Return the vegetables to the skillet, add the sauce mixture and nuts. Cook and stir over medium-high heat until thickened. Serve with rice.

BARBECUED LAMB

We often barbecue chunks of lamb with vegetables on skewers in the summer. The recipe below is very similar, but the benefit of kebabs is that you can vary the vegetables and use less meat. Vegetarian friends can also be accommodated more easily, as long as they don't mind eating from a griddle that has had meat on. The sauce is good with vegetables and I use home-grown tomatoes, baby courgettes and mushrooms as well as peppers. Use a honey and vinegar-based sauce to marinate the kebabs before cooking. They look as good as they taste.

LAMB WITH SHERRY SAUCE

You will need: Serves 6

6 lamb leg steaks
1 red pepper, cut into thick strips
1 green pepper, cut into thick strips
1 yellow pepper, cut into thick strips
120 ml (4 fluid oz) unsweetened apple juice
120 ml (4 fluid oz) honey
2 tablespoons tomato purée
2 tablespoons red wine vinegar
2 large chopped onions
2 cloves of garlic, crushed
1 teaspoon Worcestershire sauce
½ teaspoon freshly ground black pepper

Method:

1. Mix the sherry, honey, tomato purée, red wine vinegar, onion, garlic, Worcestershire sauce, pepper and apple juice in a saucepan. Simmer for 5 minutes.
2. Grill the steaks for 2 to 3 minutes, turning and brushing with the sauce. Cook with the peppers for an additional 5 minutes, or until done. Serve with a drizzle of sauce.

BRAISED PORK WITH PRUNES

You will need: Serves 4 to 5

1 kg (2 lb) boneless pork loin or shoulder
Freshly ground black pepper
2 tablespoons vegetable oil
2 onions, finely chopped
1 cinnamon stick
240 ml (8 fluid oz) chicken or vegetable stock
240 ml (8 fluid oz) water
225 g (8 oz) prunes, pitted
2 tablespoons mild honey
2 teaspoons fresh lemon juice

Method:

1. Season the meat on all sides with pepper. Brown the pork on all sides in oil in a saucepan or flameproof casserole dish over a medium-high heat. Remove the pork to a plate.

2. Stir in the onions and cook until browned. Return the pork to the pan and add any juices from the plate. Add the cinnamon, stock, and water. Bring to the boil. Reduce heat to low, cover, and simmer for 1½ hours.
Alternatively, place in a moderate oven at 180°C (350°F, gas mark 4) for the same time.
3. Add the prunes to the dish, cover, and cook until meat is very tender when pierced with a knife (about
30 minutes).
4. Stir in the honey and cook, uncovered, over low heat for 5 minutes, basting with sauce. Transfer the meat to a plate for carving and remove prunes to a bowl with a slotted spoon.
5. Boil the liquid over a high heat, stirring often, until it thickens. Add lemon juice, adjust seasoning and remove the cinnamon. Return the prunes to the casserole and reheat.
6. Arrange pork slices on a platter and spoon over the sauce and prunes.

CHINESE BEEF AND TOMATOES

You will need: Serves 6

   1 kg (2 lb) rump steak
   3 medium tomatoes
   2 green peppers
   1 tablespoon cooking oil
   2 cloves of garlic, crushed
   ¾ teaspoon fresh root ginger, finely chopped
   2 tablespoons honey
   4 tablespoons soy sauce
   1 large can bean sprouts, drained
   2 teaspoons cornflour
   4 tablespoons water
   Salt, to taste

Method:
1. Cut the steak into very thin strips. Cut tomatoes into wedges and peppers into thin strips.
2. Heat the oil in a wok or skillet. Add the beef, garlic and ginger. Stir-fry the steak over a high heat to brown. Add the honey and soy sauce, reduce heat, cover and

cook slowly for 3 to 4 minutes.
3. Add the tomatoes, peppers and bean sprouts. Cover and cook for a further 4 to 5 minutes.
4. Make a paste of cornflour and water. Add to the beef mixture and cook until the sauce thickens slightly. Add salt if required.

HONEY-GLAZED BACON

Preparing bacon or gammon with honey, mustard and cloves is a must. I use this recipe every Christmas and at other events in between. The honey gives the whole joint a wonderful glaze. Before starting, check with the supplier or on the wrapping what soaking is required, as the salt used in curing will overpower every other flavour and give you a raging thirst if you don't remove it. The bigger the joint you can manage, the better, as cold gammon will last quite a while. Well, it would in some houses anyway!

You will need: Serves 4
(modify amounts for larger joints)

    1 kg (2 lb) bacon joint, collar or gammon
    10 whole cloves
    1–2 tablespoons clear honey
    1–2 tablespoons prepared English mustard

Method:
1. Preheat the oven to 170°C (325°F, gas mark 3). Remove ham from soaking and place in a roasting tin lined with foil and covered loosely to allow air to circulate while cooking.
2. Bake for 30 minutes per lb (450 g).
3. Remove the bacon from the oven and increase the heat to 200°C (400°F, gas mark 6). Remove the rind and score the fat with a knife creating a diamond pattern. Place a clove in the centre of each diamond. Spoon the honey and mustard over the surface of the bacon. Bake in the oven for 15 minutes, basting frequently. Be careful not to allow the glaze to burn.
4. Allow to rest before carving so that the surface juices go back into the meat and it is easier to carve. If serving cold, cool thoroughly before refrigerating.

BARBECUED PORK SATÉ

This takes some time to marinate, so you need to plan ahead and prepare the day before.

You will need: Serves 6

    1 large onion, finely chopped
    1 tablespoon ground coriander
    2 tablespoons honey
    ½ teaspoon salt (adjust to taste)
    ¼ teaspoon black pepper
    1 clove of garlic, crushed
    ⅛ teaspoon cayenne pepper
    3 tablespoons fresh lemon juice
    4 tablespoons soy sauce
    650 g (1.5 lb) boneless, lean pork
    3 pitta breads, cut in half

Method:
1. Combine the first nine ingredients and cut the meat into cubes.
2. Add the meat to the marinade and mix well. Cover and refrigerate for 10 to 12 hours or overnight.
3. When ready to cook, put meat on skewers and cook over slow-burning charcoal, turning to brown on all sides. Baste often with marinade while cooking. When cooked, serve hot in pitta bread with salad.

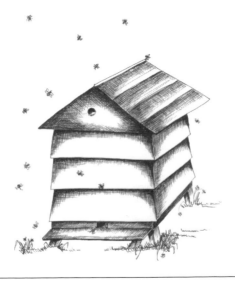

FISH DISHES

MARINATED MACKEREL

You can also use this recipe for a barbecue.

You will need: Serves 4

  2 tablespoons honey
  2 tablespoons wine vinegar
  2 tablespoons Dijon mustard
  Salt and black pepper
  4 mackerel, cleaned and boned
  4 bay leaves
  Sprigs of fresh thyme

Method:
1. Mix the honey, vinegar, mustard, salt and pepper together.
2. Place the fish in a dish, top with the bay leaves and thyme and pour over the marinade. Cover and refrigerate for 4 to 8 hours.
3. Preheat the grill, transfer the fish onto a grill rack and cook for 10 to 12 minutes, turning and basting frequently with the marinade. Serve immediately.

LINGUINE WITH PRAWNS

You will need: Serves 4

  350 g (12 oz) linguine
  2 tablespoons olive oil
  450 g (1 lb) peeled prawns (defrosted thoroughly if frozen)
  1 carrot, cut into small sticks
  1 stick celery, thinly sliced
  2 spring onions, thinly sliced on the diagonal
  2 cloves of garlic, crushed
  120 ml (4 fluid oz) water
  4 tablespoons honey
  2 teaspoons cornflour
  ¼ teaspoon cayenne pepper
  Sprig fresh rosemary or parsley
  Pinch of salt

Method:
1. Cook the linguine with salt for 8 to 10 minutes.
2. Meanwhile, heat the oil in a pan or wok, add the carrots, celery, onions and garlic, and stir-fry over a high heat for 3 to 4 minutes. Add the prawns.
3. Combine the cornflour with water, honey and pepper and add to the prawn mixture. Continue to stir-fry for 1 to 2 minutes or until sauce thickens.
4. Drain the pasta, transfer to a serving platter and pour the prawn mixture over the top. Garnish with herbs and serve immediately.

SALMON BURGERS WITH HONEY BARBECUE SAUCE

You will need: Serves 4

    4 tablespoons honey
    4 tablespoons tomato ketchup
    1 tablespoon cider vinegar
    2 teaspoons horseradish sauce
    1 clove of garlic, crushed
    1 large tin salmon, drained
    200 g (7 oz) breadcrumbs
    1 chopped onion
    1 chopped green pepper
    4 burger buns, toasted
    1 egg white

Method:
1. Combine honey, ketchup, vinegar, horseradish and garlic.
2. In a separate bowl mix together the salmon, breadcrumbs, onion, green pepper and egg white. Blend in 2 tablespoons of the sauce.
3. Divide the salmon mixture into 4, roll and flatten to make burgers. Place on a well-oiled grill or baking sheet, turning 2 to 3 times and basting with sauce, until burgers are browned and cooked through. Place on hamburger buns and serve with the rest of the sauce.

FISH WITH SWEET AND SOUR SAUCE

You will need: Serves 4

　　4 tablespoons water
　　4 tablespoons honey
　　2 tablespoons lemon juice or rice vinegar
　　2 tablespoons dry white wine
　　1 teaspoon cornflour
　　½ teaspoon garlic salt
　　1 tablespoon chopped fresh tarragon, thyme or basil
　　450 g (1 lb) fish fillets

Method:

1. Put all of the ingredients except the herbs and fish into a small saucepan. Cook over a medium heat, stirring until the mixture thickens. Simmer for 2 minutes. Add the herbs and mix well. Remove sauce from heat and keep warm.
2. Place the fish on a lightly oiled baking sheet to grill, or fry gently until the fish turns opaque and flakes easily when tested with a fork. Spoon the sauce over the fish to serve.

VEGETARIAN DISHES

BAKED HONEYED VEGETABLES

Yippee! More ways to use up a surplus of courgettes. Of course, you can vary the vegetables as you wish and as they are available. I love roasting carrots with potatoes.

You will need: Serves 4

　　12 small new potatoes, halved
　　4 tablespoons honey
　　3 tablespoons dry white wine
　　1 clove of garlic, crushed
　　Salt and pepper
　　2 teaspoons freshly chopped marjoram
　　2 courgettes, thickly sliced
　　1 small aubergine, thickly sliced
　　1 red pepper, quartered lengthways
　　1 large onion, thickly sliced
　　1 tablespoon olive oil

Method:
1. Preheat the oven to 200°C (400°F, gas mark 6).
2. Mix the honey, wine, garlic, salt, pepper and marjoram.
3. Place the vegetables in a large bowl, add the honey mixture and toss thoroughly.
4. Transfer to a shallow, oiled, ovenproof dish and bake, uncovered, for 25 minutes or until tender, mixing 2 or 3 times during the cooking period. Serve immediately.

NUT AND CARROT ROAST

You will need: Serves 4

225 g (8 oz) carrots, coarsely grated
110 g (4 oz) cashew nuts, roughly chopped
110 g (4 oz) walnut pieces
110 g (4 oz) granary breadcrumbs
50 g (2 oz) butter
1 onion, finely chopped
90 ml (3 fluid oz) vegetable stock
2 teaspoons yeast extract (Marmite)
1 teaspoon honey
1 teaspoon dried mixed herbs
2 teaspoons lemon juice
Salt and pepper

Method:
1. Preheat the oven to 180°C (350°F, gas mark 4) and grease an 850 ml (1½ pint) shallow ovenproof dish.
2. Melt the butter in a pan, add the onions and fry gently for a few minutes until soft and golden. Add the carrots and cook, stirring, for a further 5 minutes. Remove with a slotted spoon and add to the nuts and breadcrumbs in a bowl.
3. Mix the stock, yeast extract and honey in a bowl and stir until dissolved. Add to the nut mixture, together with the herbs and lemon juice. Mix well and season to taste.
4. Turn the mixture into the prepared dish and bake for 35 to 40 minutes. Serve hot or cold.

GOAT'S CHEESE PARCELS WITH
WATERCRESS SAUCE

You will need: Serves 4

    2 sheets filo pastry
    25 g (1 oz) butter, melted
    275 g (10 oz) goat's cheese
    1 bunch watercress
    240 ml (8 fluid oz) natural yoghurt
    1 teaspoon lemon juice
    1 teaspoon honey
    Salt and black pepper

Method:
1. Cut the filo pastry into 8 equal-sized squares and cover with a damp cloth to prevent them drying out while you make each parcel. Cut the goat's cheese into 4 slices.
2. Take 1 pastry square, brush with a little of the melted butter, top with another square and brush this with melted butter. Place 1 slice of goat's cheese on the pastry, gather the corners up together and pinch tightly to form a money-bag parcel. Cover with a damp cloth. Repeat with the remaining squares and cheese. Place in the fridge until you are ready to cook them.
3. Preheat the oven to 180°C, (350°F, gas mark 4).
4. Reserve 4 sprigs of the watercress and blanch the rest in boiling water for 3 minutes, or steam until wilted. Remove and drain very well, pressing as much water out as possible.
5. Place the cheese parcels on a greased baking sheet in the oven for 15 minutes
6. Place the watercress, yoghurt, honey and lemon juice in a food processor and blend until smooth. Transfer to a saucepan and warm through very gently, making sure you do not let it boil as it will curdle.
7. Divide the sauce between four serving plates, then place a parcel in the centre of the sauce and garnish with a sprig of watercress. Serve immediately.

HONEYED QUORN CHILLI

If you are not vegetarian you could substitute the quorn for lean minced beef. Alternatively, for a healthier meat option, use turkey mince, which is much better for you. I doubt if anyone will notice the difference in taste. I always use turkey mince in pasta dishes nowadays for health reasons.

You will need: Serves 6

- 1 pack quorn mince
- 1 tablespoon vegetable oil
- 1 chopped onion
- 1 chopped green pepper
- 2 cloves of garlic, finely chopped
- 1–2 tablespoons chilli powder (according to taste)
- 1 teaspoon ground cumin
- 1 teaspoon salt
- ½ teaspoon dried marjoram
- 1 large or 2 standard tins tomatoes, undrained
- 1 tin red kidney beans, washed and drained
- 2 tablespoons tomato purée
- 4 tablespoons honey
- 2 tablespoons red wine vinegar

Method:
1. In a large saucepan, heat the oil over a medium heat. Cook the onion, green pepper and garlic for 3 to 5 minutes, until the vegetables are beginning to brown.
2. Stir in the chilli powder, cumin, salt and marjoram. Stir in the quorn, cook and stir for 1 minute.
3. Stir in diced tomatoes, kidney beans, tomato purée, honey and vinegar. Bring to the boil, reduce heat and simmer, uncovered, for 15 to 20 minutes, stirring occasionally.

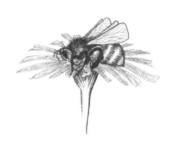

CAKES, BISCUITS AND DESSERTS

Quantities have been calculated as metric measures with imperial equivalents. As with all recipes, there may be slight variations in these amounts, so use either the metric or imperial measures, but don't mix the two.

SPICED ORANGES

You will need: Serves 4

    120 ml (4 fluid oz) red wine
    120 ml (4 fluid oz) water
    80 ml (3 fluid oz) honey
    2 whole cloves
    1 cinnamon stick
    4 slices lemon
    2 teaspoons grated orange peel
    3 navel oranges

Method:
1. Combine the wine, water, honey, spices, lemon slices and orange peel in a saucepan. Bring to the boil then reduce the heat and simmer for 15 minutes.
2. Peel the oranges and remove all white membrane. Slice the oranges thinly. Pour the hot wine syrup over the orange slices and allow to cool.
3. Cover and refrigerate for at least 4 hours. Serve in dessert dishes garnished with mint or grated dark chocolate.

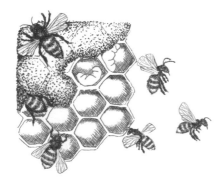

ALMOND STRAWBERRY CHEESECAKE

This recipe has the advantage of not needing to use the oven, if you plan ahead and buy a ready-made pastry shell.

You will need: Serves 6

110 g (4 oz) chocolate chips, melted
1 ready-made 22 cm (9 in) pie shell
80 ml (3 fluid oz) whipping cream
3 tablespoons honey
2 tablespoons almond-flavoured liqueur
½ teaspoon vanilla
Pinch of salt
1 punnet fresh strawberries, washed and hulled
110 g (4 oz) redcurrant jam, melted
225g (8 oz) cream cheese

Method:
1. Spread the melted chocolate over the bottom of the baked pie shell.
2. Beat the cream cheese with the whipping cream, honey, almond liqueur, vanilla and salt. Spoon over the chocolate and chill for 30 minutes.
3. Combine the strawberries with the melted jam to coat the berries. Arrange these over the cream cheese filling. Refrigerate until ready to serve.

BROWN RICE PUDDING

This has the goodness of added fibre. You can serve it with fruit such as raspberries, blueberries or even sultanas.

You will need: Serves 6

110 g (4 oz) brown rice
2 large eggs
80 ml (3 fluid oz) honey
Pinch of salt
350 ml (12 fluid oz) skimmed milk
Nutmeg or cinnamon

Method:

1. In a saucepan, bring the rice and milk to the boil. Cover, reduce heat and simmer until the rice is tender (about 45 minutes).

2. Preheat the oven to 180°C (350°F, gas mark 4). Beat together the eggs, honey and salt and stir into the hot rice.

3. Pour into a baking dish, sprinkle with nutmeg or cinnamon. Set the dish in a pan of hot water. Bake for about 50 minutes or until set. Cool. Top each serving with desired accompaniments.

FRUIT WITH HONEY LIME CREAM DRESSING

You will need: Serves 4

4 tablespoons honey
2 tablespoons lime juice
3 oranges, peeled and sliced
2 bananas, peeled and sliced
1 red apple, cored and cubed
1 green apple, cored and cubed
110 g (4 oz) shredded coconut

Method:

1. Mix the honey and lime juice and toss with the fruit. Layer fruit alternately with coconut in a serving bowl. Top with Honey Lime Cream Dressing (see below) or whipped cream.

HONEY LIME CREAM DRESSING

You will need:

120 ml (4 fluid oz) whipping cream
1 tablespoon honey
1 teaspoon grated lime peel

Method:

Beat the whipping cream until fluffy. Drizzle in the honey and beat until stiff. Fold in the grated lime peel.

DATE AND APPLE PANCAKES

If you are anything like me at making pancakes you might be inclined to buy some ready-made pancakes to fill. However, the pancakes I produced using this mixture were my best ever! If you are feeling guilty about all the forbidden goodies you've eaten, redress the balance by using wholemeal flour for the pancakes.

You will need for the pancake batter: Serves 4

    110 g (4 oz) flour
    1 egg
    275 ml (10 fluid oz) skimmed milk
    1 tablespoon oil

You will need for the filling:

    25 g (1 oz) margarine
    450 g (1 lb) eating apples, peeled, cored and chopped
    2 tablespoons honey
    ½ teaspoon mixed spice
    75 g (3 oz) chopped dates

GLAZE

You will need:

    25 g (1 oz) flaked almonds
    2 tablespoons honey

Method:

1. Put the flour in a large bowl and make a well in the middle. Add the beaten egg and gradually stir in half the milk and the oil. Beat until smooth and add the rest of the milk.

2. Heat a medium-sized frying pan and add a few drops of oil. Pour in a tablespoon of the batter and tilt the pan to coat the bottom thinly but evenly. Cook until brown and then turn and cook for another 10 seconds. Place on a warmed plate while you make the rest of the pancakes. Mine get better as I cook more.

3. Melt the margarine and cook the apples with the spice and dates for about 10 minutes, until the apples are soft. Add the honey for the filling to the pan and stir well.

4. Put some filling in each pancake and roll them and

arrange in an ovenproof dish. Warm the remaining [...] and pour over the pancakes, then sprinkle the almon[...] over the top.

5. Bake in a preheated oven for 15 minutes at 180°C (350°F, gas mark 4) and serve with crème fraîche or yoghurt.

BAKED APPLES

These are easy to prepare, delicious to eat and don't contain any fat — unless you serve them with cream.

You will need: Serves 4

  4 whole cooking apples, cored
  75 g (3 oz) dried figs, dates or raisins
  1 tablespoon honey
  1 tablespoon lemon juice
  4 tablespoons water

Method:

1. Make a cut around the middle of each apple but don't peel them. The peel will help to retain the shape. Place in an ovenproof dish with the water.

2. Push the dried fruit into the centres of the apples and pour in the lemon juice and honey.

3. Bake at 180°C (350°F, gas mark 4) for 45 to 55 minutes, until soft.

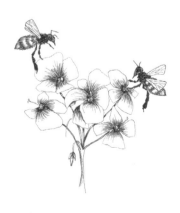

APPLE AND HONEY TART

can either make individual apple tartlets or one large
t with this recipe. If you're feeling romantic, or have
.me to kill, you can even shape the dough into hearts or
any shape you like!

You will need: Serves 6

 1 packet (approx 475 g, 1 lb) rough puff or puff pastry
 1 egg, well beaten
 240 ml (8 fluid oz) white wine or apple juice
 120 ml (4 fluid oz) honey
 1 stick cinnamon
 3 whole cloves
 1 slice fresh ginger root
 3 medium apples
 Whipped cream or crème fraîche

Method:
1. Roll the pastry out on a floured surface to a 5 mm
(¼ in) thickness. Cut one large 22 cm, (8½ in) circle,
6 x 10 cm (4 in) circles or two 12.5 cm (5 in) hearts out
of puff pastry. Cut 10 cm (½ in) wide strips of pastry from
the remaining dough. Brush the edges of the chosen
shapes with the beaten egg. Twist and line the edges with
dough strips, joining the ends with egg mixture as
necessary. Chill for 30 minutes.
2. Bake at 200°C (400°F, gas mark 6) on well-greased
baking sheets sprinkled lightly with cold water. The time
will depend on the size of the shapes, but allow 15
minutes for individual tartlets and longer for larger
shapes. When golden brown, remove or push down puffy
centres to allow space for the apple filling.
3. Bring wine or apple juice, honey and spices to the boil
in a pan, reduce heat, cover and simmer for 10 to 15
minutes. Meanwhile, peel, core and slice the apples. Add
them to the pan in one layer, and simmer until the apples
are tender but not too soft and disintegrating. Carefully
remove the slices from the liquid and drain thoroughly.
4. Reduce the liquid until syrupy and allow to cool. Brush
the bottom of the crust with syrup and arrange the
apples over the syrup. Serve with the cream.

HONEYED PLUM CRUMBLE

Crumble is a great dessert for introducing some of the less favoured but good ingredients such as oats, and for getting young people to eat fruit. I always add a spoonful or two of porridge oats to the crumble to give a nutty texture. The recipe works just as well with apples instead of plums.

You will need: Serves 4 to 6

- 900 g (2 lb) plums, halved and stoned
- 150 ml (5 fluid oz) water
- 60 ml (2 fluid oz) honey
- Juice and grated zest of an orange
- 110 g (4 oz) butter or margarine
- 225 g (8 oz) plain flour
- 50 g (2 oz) sugar
- 50 g (2 oz) toasted hazelnuts, chopped, or porridge oats

Method:

1. Preheat the oven to 200°C (400°F, gas mark 6). Place the plums, water, honey, orange juice and zest in a saucepan, bring to the boil then reduce the heat and simmer, uncovered, for 15 minutes.
2. Meanwhile, in a large mixing bowl, rub the butter or margarine into the flour with your fingertips until the mixture resembles fine breadcrumbs. Alternatively, place the whole lot into a food processor.
3. Stir in the sugar and hazelnuts, mixing well.
4. Put the plums in an ovenproof dish and sprinkle the crumble mixture evenly over the top. Bake for 35 to 40 minutes until golden. Serve hot with custard or cream.

CAKES AND BISCUITS

The moisture-absorbing qualities of honey make it a very useful aid to cooking a variety of foods and can help breads and cakes stay fresh for longer. When you substitute honey for sugar in cakes you still need to use some sugar and add a pinch of baking soda. You might also need to reduce the oven temperature slightly, to prevent overbrowning.

...cipes adapt to using honey instead of sugar in
..., as honey does not have the same properties, so
...ust be taken with cakes, otherwise they will not

HONEY CHOCOLATE CUPCAKES

You will need: Makes 12 cupcakes

50 g (2 oz) butter or margarine
180 ml (6 fluid oz) honey
1 egg
80 ml (3 fluid oz) skimmed milk
½ teaspoon vanilla extract
225 g (8 oz) plain flour
3 tablespoons unsweetened cocoa powder
¾ teaspoon baking soda
¼ teaspoon salt

Method:
1. Using an electric mixer, beat the butter until light and gradually add the honey, beating until light and creamy.
2. Beat in the egg, vanilla and milk.
3. In a separate bowl, combine the flour, cocoa, baking soda and salt, and gradually add to the butter mixture, mixing until well blended.
4. Spoon the batter into 12 paper-lined or greased muffin cups, filling each three-quarters full.
5. Bake at 180°C (350°F, gas mark 4) for 20 to 25 minutes. Remove the cakes from the oven to a wire rack and cool. Spread the top of each cupcake with chocolate icing or melted chocolate, if desired.

BAKLAVA

You will need: Makes 36 pieces

400 g (14 oz) filo pastry
350 g (12 oz) melted butter
400 g (14 oz) finely chopped almonds or walnuts
50 g (2 oz) sugar
1 teaspoon ground cinnamon
½ teaspoon ground cloves

You will need for the syrup:

    375 g (13 oz) sugar
    240 ml (8 fluid oz) honey
    Juice of 1 lemon
    360 ml (12 fluid oz) water

Method:

1. Preheat the oven to 170°C (325°F, gas mark 3) and butter two 20 x 28 cm (8 x 12 in) baking tins. Use tins that are about 5 cm (2 in) deep.

2. Mix together the nuts, sugar, cinnamon and cloves.

3. Brush 4 pieces of filo pastry with butter and place in the buttered tin, one on top of the other. (Make sure you keep the unbuttered pastry covered with a damp cloth to stop it drying out.)

4. Sprinkle the 4 sheets of pastry with a thin layer of the nut mixture, then butter two more pastry sheets and place over the top of the nut mixture. Add more of the nut mixture and then more filo pastry, until the ingredients are used up. You need to finish with 4 pastry sheets on the top.

5. Brush the top with butter and trim any edges with a sharp knife. Cut diagonally in the tin to make diamond shaped pieces, then sprinkle with water and bake for about 1 hour or until golden.

6. 10 minutes before the end of the cooking time, place the honey, water, sugar and lemon juice in a large saucepan, bring to the boil, and continue to boil for about 5 minutes. Remove the cooked baklava from the oven and pour the hot syrup evenly over the hot pastry. Cool for 10 minutes, then re-cut the diamonds. Serve warm.

BEEHIVE COOKIES

You will need:
                                      Makes approx. 30

    4 tablespoons honey
    1 egg, beaten
    1 teaspoon vanilla
    450 g (16 oz) shredded coconut
    225 g (8 oz) walnuts, coarsely chopped
    225 g (8 oz) dates, chopped
    2 tablespoons plain flour

...ogether the egg, honey and vanilla. Beat until
...ended and stir in the coconut and nuts.
...oat the dates with the flour and add to the mixture.
...Drop tablespoonfuls onto a greased baking sheet. Bake
... 170°C (325°F, gas mark 3) for 12 minutes or until
slightly brown.

HONEY AND NUT BISCUITS

You will need: Approx. 36 biscuits

110 g (4 oz) ground almonds
110 g (4 oz) ground hazelnuts
2 tablespoons honey
225 g (8 oz) caster sugar
50 g (2 oz) candied peel, chopped
2 egg whites

You will need for the icing:

4 tablespoons icing sugar
1 tablespoon lemon juice

Method:
1. Mix together all the nuts, sugar, honey, peel and egg
whites. Knead into a workable dough then leave in a cool
place for at least 30 minutes.
2. Preheat the oven to 170°C (325°F, gas mark 3) and
lightly butter and flour your baking sheets.
3. Turn the dough onto a surface dusted with icing sugar
and roll out to 5 mm (¼ in) thickness. Cut into circles, or
required shape, and transfer to the baking sheets,
allowing room to spread. Bake in the oven for 25 to
30 minutes.
4. In another bowl, mix together the icing ingredients
and use to cover the biscuits while they are still warm.
Cool completely before eating.

HONEY SHORTBREAD

You will need:

> 225 g (8 oz) butter
> 80 ml (3 fluid oz) honey
> 1 teaspoon vanilla extract
> 225 g (8 oz) plain flour
> 110 g (4 oz) finely chopped almonds

Method:

1. Preheat the oven to 150°C (300°F, gas mark 2) and lightly grease a baking tray.
2. Beat together the butter, honey and vanilla until light and fluffy. Gradually add the flour and almonds and mix well.
3. Turn onto a lightly floured board and knead lightly to about 10 mm (½ in) thickness, to fit the shape of your baking sheet. Transfer to the baking tray and mark into slices with a knife. Bake for 40 minutes. Transfer to a wire rack to cool.

HONEY FLAPJACKS

You will need:

> 200 g (7 oz) butter
> 200 g (7 oz) demerara sugar
> 200 g (7 oz) honey
> 400 g (14 oz) porridge oats
> 50 g (2 oz) nuts, dried fruits, glacé cherries,
>   chopped or desiccated coconut (optional)

Method:

1. Heat the butter, sugar and honey until the sugar has dissolved.
2. Add the oats and nuts, fruit or coconut and mix well.
3. Place in a greased Swiss roll tin or cake tin and spread to about 2 cm (¾ in) thick.
4. Bake in a preheated oven at 180°C (350°F, gas mark 4) for 15 to 20 minutes, until golden around the edges, but soft in the middle. Let it cool in the tin, then turn out and cut into squares.

KHUBS (MOROCCAN BREAD)

You will need: Makes 1 round loaf
1 teaspoon honey
360 ml (12 fluid oz) lukewarm water
1 tablespoon dried yeast
1½ teaspoons salt
450 g (1 lb) strong plain white flour

Method:
1. Lightly flour a baking tray and set aside. In a small bowl, mix together the water, honey and yeast and allow to stand for 10 minutes.
2. In a large bowl, mix together the flour and salt. Make a well in the centre and pour in the yeast mixture. Mix to form a firm dough before transferring to a floured surface. Knead for about 5 minutes.
3. Form the dough into a round loaf, place on the baking tray and cover with a plastic bag or clean tea towel. Leave in a warm place to rise, until it doubles in size (about 30 minutes).
4. Preheat the oven to 190°C (375°F, gas mark 5). Knead the loaf lightly and transfer it to the oven. Bake it for about 45 minutes. Allow to cool before serving.

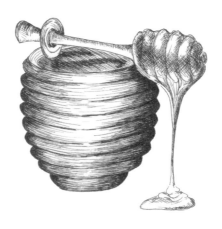

CRANBERRY AND HONEY OAT BREAD

You will need: Makes 1 loaf

2 tablespoons honey
1 egg
175 ml (6 fluid oz) milk
1 teaspoon melted butter or margarine
350 g (12 oz) plain flour
175 g (6 oz) rolled (porridge) oats
1 dessertspoon baking powder
½ teaspoon salt
½ teaspoon ground cinnamon
110 g (4 oz) fresh or frozen cranberries
50 g (2 oz) chopped nuts (optional)

Method:

1. Preheat the oven to 180°C (350°F, gas mark 4) and grease a loaf tin.
2. Put the flour, oats, baking powder and salt in a bowl.
3. Beat together the egg, honey and milk and add to the flour and oats, stirring well. Fold in the cranberries and nuts.
4. Pour into the loaf tin and bake for about 75 minutes, or until crusty and hollow when knocked. Pour the melted butter over the hot loaf and turn out onto a cooling rack.

FROZEN DESSERTS

You don't need an ice cream maker to achieve good results with home-made ice cream, although it may take some of the effort out. The good thing about making your own is that you can amend the recipes to suit healthy options and avoid too much sugar. Ice cream is rarely made entirely of cream. You can use equal parts of cream and custard, cream and fruit purée, cream and egg whites, or replace the cream with unsweetened evaporated milk or plain yoghurt. The cream can be double, whipping or a low fat blend of buttermilk and vegetable oils, such as Elmlea.

HONEY AND RASPBERRY ICE CREAM

You will need:

    450 g (1 lb) raspberries
    150 ml (¼ pint) cream
    150 ml (¼ pint) plain yoghurt
    3 egg whites
    2 tablespoons lemon juice
    10 level tablespoons honey
    Pinch of salt

Method:

1. Sieve the raspberries to give you a purée and blend with the cream, yoghurt, lemon juice, honey and salt. Put this mix into a shallow plastic container and freeze until firm, but not totally frozen.

2. Return to a bowl and beat until smooth. Whisk the egg whites until stiff and fold into the ice cream. Return to the tray and freeze.

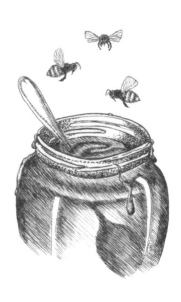

FROZEN HONEY YOGHURT

You will need:

570 ml (1 pint) skimmed milk
200 ml (7 fluid oz) honey
Pinch of salt
2 eggs, beaten
500 g (17½ oz) (large) pot plain low-fat yoghurt
1 tablespoon vanilla essence

Method:

1. Heat the milk in a large saucepan but don't boil it. Stir in the honey and salt.
2. Pour a small amount of milk mixture into the eggs and then return to the remaining milk mixture in the saucepan. Cook and stir over medium-low heat for 5 minutes or until the mixture coats the back of a wooden spoon. Do not boil.
3. Remove from the heat and cool completely. Stir in the yoghurt and vanilla and turn into a plastic dish. Freeze until firm, stirring every 20 to 30 minutes to break up the ice crystals, or freeze in an ice cream maker, according to manufacturer's directions.

FROZEN NECTARINE YOGHURT

You will need: Serves 6

5 ripe nectarines, peeled and chopped
240 ml (8 fluid oz) water
4 tablespoons honey
1 tablespoon lemon juice
1 teaspoon vanilla
4 tablespoons apple juice
225 g (8 oz) plain low-fat yoghurt

Method:

1. Put the nectarines, water and honey in a saucepan and cook over medium heat until the nectarines are soft. Purée them in a blender.
2. Stir in the lemon juice, vanilla and apple juice. Chill until cool.

hisk the yoghurt into the nectarine mixture. Pour
a freezable dish and freeze until crystals form
und the edges (about 45 minutes). Stir the crystals
to the middle of the pan and return to freezer. When
lightly frozen through, whip again and refreeze.

BEE BERRY SORBET

Sorbet differs from ice cream in that it is a semi-frozen
ice based dessert; much lower in calories without the
cream or yoghurt.

You will need: Serves 6

  450 g (1 lb) raspberries
  4 tablespoons honey
  4 tablespoons fresh lime juice, including pulp
  ¼ teaspoon grated lime peel
  240 ml (8 fluid oz) water

Method:
1. Purée the raspberries and sieve to remove the pips.
Add the remaining ingredients and mix well.
2. Pour into a freezer-safe dish and freezer for 3 to 6
hours or until firm.
3. Transfer the mixture to a bowl. Beat with an electric
mixer until slushy but not thawed. Return to the dish and
freeze for 2 to 4 hours, or until firm.

Fascinating
Facts
& Appendices

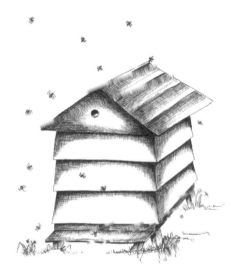

THE BEES ARE BUZZING OFF

A jumbo jet heading from Sydney to London was diverted to a tiny landing strip at Uralsk in Kazakhstan, when a fire hazard light was set off. Sensors suggested a fire in the cockpit, but all that could be found was a package of angry bees en route for Britain. It took 20 hours to ferry passengers back to London in smaller craft, as the airstrip was too short for the jumbo to take off with its passengers on board. All because of a bunch of bothered bees.

BEE STATISTICS

• Bees fly 55,000 miles to make a pound of honey. That's the equivalent of one and a half times around the world.

• To make a pound of beeswax a bee needs 2.7 kg (6 lb) of honey.

• The average hive produces 11 kg (25 lb) of honey per year. One hive can produce 27 kg (60 lb) in a good season.

• Rob Smith, an Australian bee-keeper, produced a world record 346 kg (762 lb) from each of 460 hives in 1954.

BE(E)HAVE YOURSELF!

CHARLES HENRY TURNER
Dr Turner was the first African-American to earn a Ph.D. at the University of Chicago in about 1890. His work on the colour-vision of bees and their recognition of patterns and shapes and his ability to time bees' appearance for feedings pre-dated von Frisch's similar work.

KARL VON FRISCH
This German scientist interpreted the bees' waggle dance. For this and his other, related animal behaviour studies, he won the Nobel Prize.

FRANÇOIS HUBER
In the late 18th century, the blind Swiss naturalist and bee-keeper Huber developed special beehives, to improve scientific observation of his bees. His work, viewed through the eyes of his assistant, resulted in the first clear understanding of the concept of 'bee space', leading to the building of modern hives with movable frames.

FAMOUS CENTENARIANS

DEMOCRITUS
This Greek apicultural researcher, bee-keeper and philosopher, who apparently lived to the great age of 109, taught that new bees could be made from rotting oxen. Well he couldn't be right all of the time . . .

FRED HALE
Before he died, aged 113, in November 2004, Maine bee-keeper Fred Hale was the oldest (documented) man in the world. He was driving a car at age 107 and shovelling snow at 112.

ROMAN EMPEROR AUGUSTUS
Augustus asked a centenarian how he had lived to be 100. The reply he received gave food for thought:

'Oil without and honey within.'

MONASTIC BEES

ABBÉ COLLIN
This French bee-keeper invented the queen excluder in 1865.

GREGOR MENDEL
Gregor Mendel, a monk, was the father of genetics. A keen bee-keeper, Mendel discovered the fundamental laws of genetics in pea plants, then spent the rest of his life trying to breed better bees, without success.

CARL KEHRLE
Also known as Brother Adam, this Benedictine monk developed the Buckfast Abbey bee in 1917 and became renowned worldwide for his scientific research into bee breeding.

STAR QUALITY HONEY

HENRY FONDA
Hollywood legend and star of 96 films, this hobby bee-keeper gave away honey in jars that he labelled 'Henry's Honey'.

PETER FONDA
Peter Fonda, son of Henry, actor and activist, was named Bee-keeper of the Year by the Florida State Bee-keeping Association for deftly portraying Ulee in 'Ulee's Gold', and for his contribution to bee-keeping.

PHILOSOPHICAL HONEY

HIPPOCRATES
The father of medicine frequently recommended honey as a remedy for whatever ailed patients. He wrote, 'Honey and pollen cause warmth, clean sores and ulcers, soften hard ulcers of lips, heal carbuncles and running sores.'

MARCUS AURELIUS
This famous Roman emperor, philosopher, and potentially the world's first Socialist said, 'What is not good for the swarm is not good for the bee.'

CLIMB EVERY MOUNTAIN . . .

SIR EDMUND HILLARY
The son of a New Zealand commercial bee-keeper, Hillary and his brother owned 1,200 hives. Along with Tenzing Norgay, he first scaled Mount Everest in May 1953. He then gave up bee-keeping in favour of mountaineering.

MARIA VON TRAPP
After the family escaped from wartime Austria, this ex-nun and governess moved to Vermont and kept bees.

POLITICAL LEADERS

LYCURGUS
The founder of Sparta was much impressed by the honey bees' social structure, sacrifice, and sharing. He used the bee colony as a model for a perfect form of government.

NAPOLEON BONAPARTE
'Boney' used the bee as a personal symbol of his immortality. His red cape is remembered for its bee print.

VIKTOR YUSHCHENKO
The leader of the democracy movement and president of the Ukraine is an avid bee-keeper.

DAN QUAYLE
The former US vice-president's response to bee-keepers seeking price-support help was: 'Bee-keeping is a sweet subsidy that has been ripping off taxpayers for years.' Not a fan, then!

THE GREAT AND THE GODS

ALEXANDER THE GREAT
When the great conqueror died thousands of miles from home, his men carried his preserved body home for burial in a golden coffin filled with honey.

RAMESES III
This ancient Egyptian pharaoh, king and deity from 1198 to 1167 BC, offered a lesser river god a 30,000 lb honey sacrifice by dumping honey into the Nile.

ICARUS
The ancient astronaut of Greek mythology flew too close to the sun and the beeswax holding the feathers to his arms melted and came loose. Legend has it that he is still falling.

AGAINST IDLENESS AND MISCHIEF

How doth the little busy bee
Improve each shining hour,
And gather honey all the day
From every shining flower!

How skilfully she builds her cell!
How neat she spreads the wax!
And labours hard to store it well
With the sweet food she makes.

This excerpt from a poem by Isaac Watts was parodied by
Lewis Carroll in *Alice in Wonderland*.

I eat my peas with honey,
I've done it all my life,
It makes the peas taste funny,
But it keeps them on the knife.

Anon

The pedigree of honey
Does not concern the bee,
A clover, any time, to him,
Is aristocracy.

Emily Dickinson

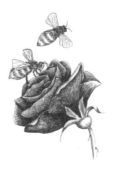

PROVERBS

More flies are taken with a drop of honey than
a Tun of Vinegar.

Thomas Fuller, 1732

When you shoot an arrow of truth,
dip its point in honey.

Arab proverb

Life is the flower of which love is the honey.

Victor Hugo

Lovers, like bees,
lead a honey sweet life.

Graffiti found in Pompeii

HYDROMEL, OR HONEY WINE: FROM 'THE CLOSET OF SIR KENELM DIGBY, KNIGHT, OPENED 1699'

'Take 18 quarts of spring water and one quart of honey: when the water is warm, put the honey into it. When it boileth up, skim it very well and continue skimming it, as long as any scum will rise. Then put in one race [root] of Ginger, four Cloves and a little sprig of Rosemary. Let these boil in the Liquor so long, till in all it have boiled one hour. Then set it to cool, till it be blood-warm, and then put to it a spoonful of Ale-yeast. When it is worked up, put it into a vessel of a fit size: and after two to three days, bottle it up. You may drink it after six weeks or two months.

This was the hydromel that I gave the Queen, which was exceedingly liked by everybody.'

APPENDIX 1

LIST OF HONEYS

Acacia
Alfalfa
Apple blossom
Aster
Athel tree
Avocado
Bamboo
Basswood
Bergamot
Blackberry
Blue curis
Blue gum
    (Eucalyptus)
Blueberry
Bluevine
Boneset
Buckwheat
Cantaloupe
Cape vine
Cherry blossom
Chestnut
Chinquapin
Clover
Coralvine
Coriander
Cotton
Cranberry
Eucalyptus
Fireweed
Gallberry
Golden rod

Grape
Hawthorn
Hedysarum
    Coronarium
Holly
Iron bark
    (Eucalyptus)
Horeminy
Kamahi
Lavender
Leatherwood
Lime blossom
Locust
Manuka
Manzanita
Marigold
Mesquite
Mexican clover
Mint
Mountain laurel
Mustard
Nodding thistle
Orange
Orange blossom
Palmetto
Pepperbush
Peppermint
Peppervine
Poison oak
Poplar
Privet

Prune
Raspberry
Rata
Rewarewa
River red gum
    (Eucalyptus)
Sage
Sea lavender
Snowbush
Sourwood
Soybean
Spanish needle
Spearmint
Star thistle
Strawberry tree
Stringybark
    (Eucalyptus)
Sumac
Sunflower
Tawari
Thistle
Thyme
Titi
Trefoil
Tulip tree
Tupelo
Viper's bugloss
Yellow box
    (Eucalyptus)

APPENDIX 2

SOME MAJOR SOURCES OF NECTAR IN THE NORTHERN HEMISPHERE

Alfalfa
Apple blossom
Aster
Basswood
Blackberry
Blackthorn
Clover
Dandelion
Field beans

Fireweed
Globe thistle
Golden rod
Heather
Knapweed
Lavender
Milkweed
Oilseed rape
Pussy willow

Raspberry
Rosebay
    willowherb
Sea lavender
Smartweed
Soybean
Sumac
Willow